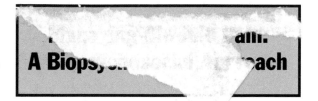

A Biops... ...ach

£29.28

Managing Chronic Pain: A Biopsychosocial Approach

SAXBY PRIDMORE, MB, BS, BMEDSC, DPHYSIO, MD
FRANZCP, FAFPHM
CLINICAL PROFESSOR OF PSYCHIATRY
UNIVERSITY OF TASMANIA
AND
DIRECTOR OF PSYCHOLOGICAL MEDICINE
ROYAL HOBART HOSPITAL
TASMANIA, AUSTRALIA

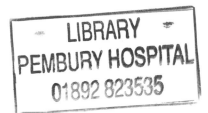
MARTIN DUNITZ

© 2002 Martin Dunitz Ltd, a member of the Taylor & Francis group

First published in the United Kingdom in 2002 by Martin Dunitz Ltd,
The Livery House, 7–9 Pratt Street, London NW1 0AE

Tel: +44 (0) 20 7482 2202
Fax: +44 (0) 20 7267 0159
E-mail: info@dunitz.co.uk
Webiste: http://www.dunitz.co.uk

A CIP record for this book is available from the British Library.

ISBN 1 84184 162 5

Distributed in the USA by
Fulfilment Center
Taylor & Francis
7625 Empire Drive
Florence, KY 41042, USA
Toll Free Tel.: +1 800 634 7064
E-mail: cserve@routledge_ny.com

Distributed in Canada by
Taylor & Francis
74 Rolark Drive
Scarborough, Ontario M1R 4G2, Canada
Toll Free Tel.: +1 877 226 2237
E-mail: tal_fran@istar.ca

Distributed in the rest of the world by
ITPS Limited
Cheriton House
North Way
Andover, Hampshire SP10 5BE, UK
Tel.: +44 (0)1264 332424
E-mail: reception@itps.co.uk

Composition by Wearset Ltd, Boldon, Tyne and Wear
Printed and bound by Gutenberg Press Ltd, Malta

Contents

Said a faith-healer from Brazil
'I know that pain isn't real
but when I sit on a pin
and it pricks my skin
I dislike what I fancy I feel.'
                                    Anonymous

Introduction

'To help the patient to cope the psychiatrist must be a teacher, doctor, soothsayer, and wise friend with the right mixture of palliative care, hope, denial, catharsis, family counseling, relaxation, exercise, physical rehabilitation, pharmacotherapy, and sensitivity to the unconscious.'

Anthony Bouckoms, 1996

Pain is a common human experience, but difficult to describe. The most influential definition (Merskey, 1979) states that pain is an unpleasant sensory and emotional experience that is associated with actual tissue damage or is described in terms of such damage. Immediately, unexpected elements are introduced by this definition: pain involves an emotional experience; and it may be experienced in the absence of 'actual' tissue damage.

Acute pain is a component of the warning system that helps to preserve the individual and the species. Nociceptors are specific primary afferent nerves that respond to potentially tissue-damaging stimuli. Nociception is the activity in the nervous system that occurs as a consequence of nociceptor stimulation. A physiological view is that pain is the perception of nociception. However, it is more than sensory system activity. Nociception, through identified hard-wired circuits, triggers emotional and motivational-affective responses (which can be called the pain experience). The environmental circumstances that give rise to the nociception, along with the acute pain experience, are stored in memory. Thus, not only can the circumstances that lead to danger be avoided in the future (providing survival advantage), but the pain experience can be remembered in the future, providing at least a partial basis for chronic pain.

In addition to the acute–chronic division, pain can be classified according to current pathophysiologic knowledge. This introduces nociceptive, neuropathic and psychogenic pain. Nociceptive pain occurs when the nervous system is intact and the symptoms are consistent with known or suspected somatic or visceral damage. Neuropathic pain is the result of an abnormality of the nervous system. A range of pathophysiological mechanisms may be present in the peripheral, central or sympathetic systems. The term 'psychogenic pain' has been applied when psychological factors appear to be of primary aetiological importance (Roth, 2000).

Often the tissues producing nociceptive pain (a calf muscle injury, for example) heal in a matter of weeks and the pain resolves. Where this does not happen there is usually an ongoing process, such as an inflammatory or a neoplastic process, and specialists experienced in the management of this

symptom (rheumatologists, oncologists) provide direction. The neuropathic and psychogenic chronic pain syndromes are less well understood and managed. Other important chronic pain syndromes include fibromyalgia and the various headaches, which may involve complicated mixtures of physical and psychological contributions.

Chronic pain lacks a useful function. It has been defined as pain lasting more than six weeks (Bouckoms, 1996) and as pain lasting more than six months (Russo & Brose, 1998). Others (Loeser and Melzack, 1999) have argued for a conceptual rather than a quantitative definition: 'It is not the duration of pain that distinguishes acute from chronic pain but, more importantly, the inability of the body to restore its physiological functions to normal homeostatic levels.'

Chronic pain is a common disorder that causes great individual suffering. It is costly in fiscal as well as human terms. It is often associated with increasing dependence, irritability, somatic concern, social withdrawal, physical and occupational disability, and a higher than normal prevalence of psychiatric disorders such as anxiety and depression.

Non-invasive techniques such as provision of information, goal setting, pharmacotherapy, relaxation, logical thinking, and exploration of psychological issues are important in chronic pain reduction. In many cases they constitute the most appropriate approach. In other cases they are an alternative to the invasive therapeutic techniques. When the invasive therapeutic techniques are the treatment of choice, the addition of complementary non-invasive techniques ensures comprehensive care.

Invasive techniques in chronic pain comprise an array of diagnostic and therapeutic manoeuvres that rest on an extensive scientific base. It is unreasonable to expect invasive therapeutic techniques to bring relief if the evidence for a treatable organic pathology is doubtful or when similar past treatments have brought little lasting relief.

The biopsychosocial model of illness, which emphasizes the contribution of biological/medical, psychological/psychiatric and social/environmental factors in aetiology and management, has been a guiding concept in psychiatry and comprehensive family medicine for more than two decades. It is the ideal recommended approach in all forms of pain (Cheville et al, 2000). The social/environmental component should be expanded to include cultural factors. Different ethnic groups demonstrate different responses to the experience of pain (Zborowski, 1969), and it is argued that 'pain and suffering in society are manifested in pain and suffering in the body' (Ware and Kleinman, 1992).

This book contains theoretical and practical information that will assist a range of professionals in their work with patients with chronic pain. A particular aim is to provide material that will be useful to Psychiatrists and General Practitioners.

References

Bouckoms A. Chronic pain: neuropsychopharmacology and adjunctive psychiatric treatment. In: Rundell J, Wise M (eds) *Textbook of Consultation-Liaison Psychiatry.* American Psychiatric Press, Washington, DC, 1996; 1007–36.

Cheville A, Caaceni A, Portney R. Pain: definition and assessment. In: Massie MJ (ed) *Pain: What Psychiatrists Need to Know.* (Review of Psychiatry Series, Vol. 19, No 2; Oldham J and Riba M, series eds). American Psychiatric Press, Washington, DC, 2000; 1–22.

Loeser J, Melzack R. Pain: an overview. *Lancet* 1999; 353: 1607–9.

Merskey H. Pain terms: a list with definitions and a note on usage. Recommended by the International Association for the Study of Pain (IASP) Subcommittee on Taxonomy. *Pain* 1979; 6: 249–52.

Roth R. Psychogenic models of chronic pain: a selective review and critique. In: Massie MJ (ed) *Pain: What Psychiatrists Need to Know.* (Review of Psychiatry Series, Vol. 19, No 2; Oldham J and Riba M, series eds). American Psychiatric Press, Washington, DC, 2000; 89–131.

Russo C, Brose W. Chronic pain. *Annual Review of Medicine* 1998; 49: 123–33.

Ware N, Kleinman A. Culture and somatic experience: the social course of illness in neurasthenia and chronic fatigue syndrome. *Psychosomatic Medicine* 1992; 54: 546–60.

Zborowski M. *People in Pain.* Jossey-Bass, San Francisco, 1969.

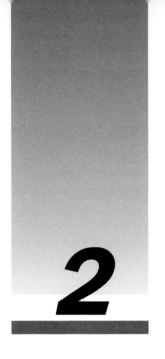

A reasonable approach to chronic pain reduction

2

'Doctors think a lot of patients are cured who have simply quit in disgust.'

Don Herold

Woven together, the following points form a useful approach to chronic pain.

1. The fundamental Hippocratic principle of 'first do no harm' applies throughout medical practice. In chronic pain management, the non-invasive techniques carry a low risk of causing harm. There is a need to prescribe medication cautiously and to make every effort to avoid medication abuse and addiction.

2. Comprehensive examination and investigation is mandatory. Once this process is complete the most likely diagnosis should be decided and the most appropriate treatment commenced. It is not necessary for the pain therapists to re-investigate the case, if suitable investigations have already been conducted by a capable clinician. Further investigations should be kept to a minimum and should be conducted only when there is good reason to expect that the result will be different from those obtained previously.

3. The health professionals working in chronic pain should communicate that they accept that the patient's pain is 'real'. This is the case in all except malingerers. Research has revealed a range of mechanisms by which firing thresholds of sensory processing neurones may be lowered, allowing for stronger pain than might have been expected in particular clinical situations. Pain that is predominantly of psychological origin is no less real to the patient than that which is predominantly of physical origin.

4. A supportive patient–therapist relationship is encouraged. The characteristics of this relationship differ slightly, depending on the theoretical and clinical training of the therapist. Universal characteristics are respect for the patient and the belief that patient choices are possible and change is necessary.

5. Pain is best conceptualized using the biopsychosocial model. Thus, both biological/physical, psychological/psychiatric and social/environmental factors should be considered in both aetiology and treatment.

6. Whenever possible, a person from the patient's family or social life should be involved in the examination and treatment process. This may be a partner, relative or friend. Such an individual can give important information regarding the patient's level of function in daily life and encourage the patient to comply with professional suggestions when at home or in social settings.

7. It is most important to provide the patient with good information, from the first and at every subsequent meeting.

8. Realistic expectations should be encouraged. Chronic pain has by definition persisted well beyond the normal healing time. It is realistic to expect that treatment will reduce pain and make a fuller life possible (albeit with residual pain). While it is healthy to hope and work toward complete cessation of pain, it is also healthy for the patient to understand and accept that this may be unlikely given present medical knowledge and technology. Accordingly, in most cases it is unhealthy, in so far as it will delay adjustment and risk iatrogenic complications, for patients to persist in the search for the total medical cure to chronic pain.

9. Patients need to be prepared for setbacks. Fluctuations in clinical state are a feature of all chronic conditions. These are particularly common when activity is increased. Patients who are increasing their activity after a period of relative inactivity need to expect such

fluctuations and to continue (rather than abandon) the pain reduction process.

10. Hurting does not indicate harm. In chronic pain there has been time for the healing of any damaged structures. Unstable joints will have been stabilized, entrapped structures will have been released and any other necessary procedures will have been performed. Thus, pain associated with activity does not indicate further damage to the body. It is most important for the patient to understand and accept this point.

11. Return to normal or near-normal activity is desirable. Pain fosters inactivity. This results in loss of motor power and joint stiffness. As muscles atrophy they lose the capacity to perform their 'bracing' or supporting function. Thus pain and inactivity can lead to the downward spiral of ever more pain and inactivity. Inactivity has the additional unhelpful consequence of loss of social role and self-esteem. Retaining or returning to near-normal activity minimizes pain and provides a range of benefits.

12. Operant conditioning-based therapy states that the rewarding of positive efforts with encouragement and the non-rewarding of (withholding of approval from) pain behaviour may encourage return to normal behaviour. The weakness of behaviourism in this clinical setting is that pain is not simply a pattern of behaviour. It is also an experience. Nevertheless, it makes sense to encourage behaviour that does not typify the patient as an invalid.

13. Operant formulations that pain behaviour is performed as a means of attracting rewards lead to scepticism and suspicion of malingering. It may result in unfair withholding of support. The apparent increase in pain behaviour when a patient is in the presence of supportive individuals is given a different and more positive interpretation by evolutionary psychology. The patient is viewed as suppressing or hiding pain behaviour when in the company of unsupportive individuals 'in the field'; however, in supportive environments, this suppression is released and pain behaviour, vulnerability and care-eliciting are revealed.

14. Pacing behaviour is encouraged. Clinical wisdom is that when patients with chronic pain have relatively pain-free periods, they tend to be overactive, which then causes temporary increases in pain. These 'flare ups' result in a return to periods of inactivity. Instead, patients are encouraged to 'pace' themselves: to be active regularly, but to limit the amount of activity so that 'flare ups' do not occur. Specific studies to support 'pacing' have not been reported, but the concept has face validity.

15. Logical thinking is more helpful than illogical thinking. Thoughts influence the way one feels. This is the basis of the original cognitive behaviour therapy. Thoughts such as 'I cannot pick my children up so I am a failure as a parent' result in demoralization and depression, and must be challenged and corrected for the patient to achieve the best possible result.

16. Relaxation training, self-hypnosis and medication have all been shown to relieve chronic pain. The patient should be taught and encouraged to practise at least one such technique.

17. Psychotherapy has a place when there is a need for the patient to adjust human relationships, sense of self or goals. It is particularly indicated where psychological factors are important in the aetiology or maintenance of pain. It may also be indicated where physically based pain necessitates difficult psychological adjustments.

18. Medication is indicated, almost without exception. Excessive or inappropriate medication, however, is to be avoided. This is particularly the case with the short-acting opioids and certain benzodiazepines. Such medications have limited beneficial effects in chronic pain and carry the risk of addiction.

19. Excessive health-care utilization is discouraged. It not only wastes the patient's resources and delays recovery, but is also wasteful of community resources. It usually arises from excessive patient concern about the pain. Reducing undue utilization is not an easy task and may, after clear and repeated reassurance and a period of support, call for limit-setting.

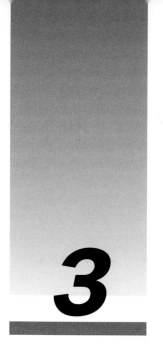

Anatomy and physiology

3

'Symptoms, then, are in reality nothing but the cry from suffering organs.'

Jean-Martin Charcot

The anatomic and physiologic basis of pain is a highly sophisticated and emerging field. The interested reader should consult encyclopaedic textbooks such as Bonica (1990a), Wall and Melzack (1999) and Haines (1997).

Most clinicians do not require the details of latest animal laboratory studies. Instead, a brief account is presented that brings some preclinical and clinical matters together.

Local response to trauma/inflammation

Initial traumatic events depolarize pain neurones and cause initial pain. Subsequent physiologic changes make these neurones more sensitive than normal to noxious stimuli (hyperalgesia).

The macroscopic hallmarks of trauma/inflammation are redness, swelling, heat and loss of function (which encourages repair). The microscopic hallmark is the accumulation of fluid and cells at the site. Mast cells are important activators, releasing histamine from preformed cytoplasmic granules and synthesizing other mediators, including prostaglandins. Serotonin is produced by platelets. Bradykinin is synthesized in the plasma. Substance P (sP) is released from stimulated nerve endings. Catecholamines are released from sympathetic endings into the traumatized region.

Histamine, prostaglandins, serotonin, bradykinin, sP and catecholamines, among other agents, are believed to increase the permeability of capillaries, resulting in the local swelling. Also, they excite pain neurones and are responsible for the hyperalgesia.

Primary sensory neurones

There are two broad groups of sensory neurones: (1) myelinated A fibres, and (2) smaller diameter, unmyelinated C fibres.

A-beta fibres have a low threshold and transmit non-noxious tactile and mechanical information.

Thinly myelinated A-delta fibres and C fibres have a higher threshold and are nociceptors: specific primary sensory neurones that signal noxious stimulation. They are activated by energy (mechanical, thermal or chemical), which can, in the extreme, cause tissue damage.

A-delta fibres detect mechanical and thermal stimuli. They transmit impulses rapidly (12–30 m/s) and provide the 'first pain'. C fibres are 'polymodal', responding to

a range of stimuli. They transmit slowly (1 m/s) and provide the 'slow pain', which is felt 1–2 s after the application of a noxious stimulus.

Terminals of the primary afferents

There is some individual variation in the arrangement of the neural structures subserving pain. Thus, predictions of aetiology and response to procedures should be attempted with caution. The following is the most common arrangement (see Figure 3.1):

Sensory neurones have cell bodies in the dorsal root ganglion and enter the spinal cord via the dorsal root. They divide into ascending and descending branches and travel short distances in the dorsolateral tract before terminating in the dorsal horn. The dorsal horn is arranged in a series of laminae (Brose and Spiegel, 1992).

Lamina I is superficial and posteriorly located. The second-order neurones with cell bodies in this lamina receive input from nociceptors A-delta and C fibres.

Lamina II is deep to lamina I and is known as substantia gelatinosa, on the basis of its appearance. The second-order neurones in this lamina receive input exclusively from C fibres (Woolf and Mannion, 1999). In addition, lamina II is densely packed with small cells that synapse both internally and in

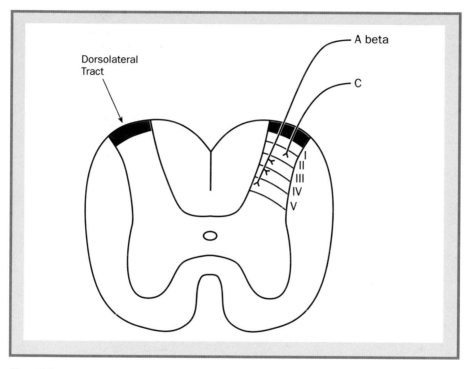

Figure 3.1
Termination of peripheral sensory neurones in the laminae of the dorsal horn (much simplified). Touch (A beta) fibres terminate in lamina III, IV or V. Pain (C) fibres terminate predominantly in lamina II. The dorsolateral tract is superficial to laminae I and II.

other laminae. They are important in the inhibition of second-order cells.

Laminae III and IV contain the cell bodies of neurones that receive the terminal projections of A-beta neurones, which are responsive to non-noxious stimulation, including touch.

Ascending sensory pathways

The axons of the second-order cells of the dorsal horn usually cross the cord and pass upward as the spinothalamic or spinoreticular systems (see Figures 3.2 and 3.3), within the contralateral anterolateral funiculus (Price, 2000). The spinothalamic system is composed of neospinothalamic and palaeospinothalamic divisions.

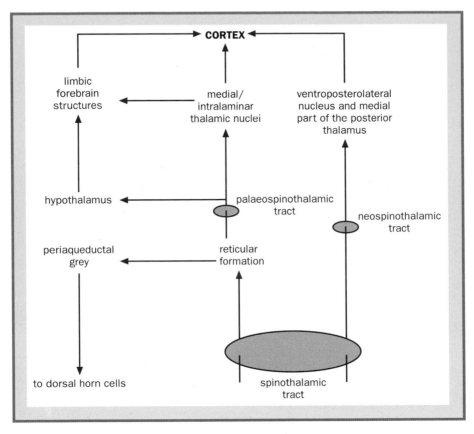

Figure 3.2
Projection of spinothalamic tract. The spinothalamic tract (composed of palaeospinothalamic and neospinothalamic fibres) is passing upward at the bottom right.

The fibres which are to become the palaeospinothalamic tract relay at the reticular formation. Projections then proceed to the hypothalamus and thalamus, and subsequently, the limbic system and cortex. This arrangement may provide the anatomical substrate for the emotional and motivational aspects of pain. The neospinothalamic tract bypasses the reticular formation and relays at the thalamus before reaching the cortex. It is believed to provide an anatomical substrate for the informational aspects of pain. Projections from the reticular formation to the periaqueductal grey matter are part of a feedback pathway to the dorsal horn cells.

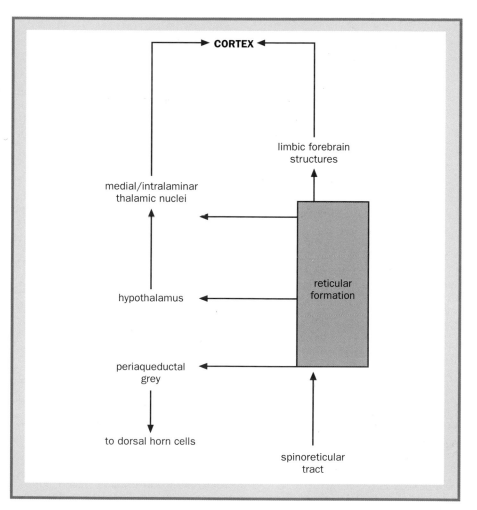

Figure 3.3
Projections of spinoreticular tract. The spinoreticular tract is passing upward at the bottom right. It ends at the reticular formation. Output from the reticular formation goes to the hypothalamus, thalamus and the limbic system. Projections then reach the cortex. This arrangement may provide the anatomical substrate for the emotional and motivational aspects of pain in the human.

As with the spinothalamic tract, output from the reticular formation goes to the periaqueductal grey matter which projects to the dorsal horn cells, thus providing a mechanism for the reduction of nociceptive input.

Other ascending nociceptive pathways are found in the spinomesencephalic tract, dorsal column system, spinocervical tract and multisynaptic ascending system (Bonica, 1990b). These are listed only and will not be discussed further.

Brain-stem relays

The brain stem contains a complex arrangement of grey matter nuclei. Most pathways, passing in both directions (cephalad and caudad), synapse in the brain stem and can be modified at these relay stations. (The neospinothalamic tract bypasses these nuclei, and is thus an exception.)

The reticular formation extends from the mesencephalon through the pons to the medulla. It is described as a collection of nineteen separate nuclei (Bonica, 1990b); but for simplicity, it can be considered here as a single entity. In this view the important locus coeruleus is an integral part of the reticular formation. The reticular formation projects fibres to the thalamus, hypothalamus and limbic structures.

The periaqueductal grey matter is situated in the midbrain. Along with the locus coeruleus and other reticular formation nuclei, it has an important role in modifying descending information, both locally and via projections that descend in the dorsal columns to the dorsal horn cells at segmental levels.

Thalamus

The thalamus is a complex of many nuclei, differently named by different authors. For present purposes, we can focus on two parts: (1) the posterior thalamus (precisely, the ventroposterolateral thalamic nucleus, and the medial part of the posterior thalamus); and (2) the medial/intralaminar thalamic nuclei.

The posterior thalamus receives input from the neospinothalamic tract, which bypasses the reticular formation. It projects to the cortex.

The medial/intralaminar thalamic nuclei receive pathways from the reticular formation, which is a relay station of the palaeospinothalamic and the spinoreticular tracts.

The medial/intralaminar thalamic nuclei nociceptive outflows go to the hypothalamus, limbic forebrain structures and the cerebral cortex. The connections with the limbic system are believed to provide the mechanism for the emotional and motivational aspects of pain.

The cortex

The posterior thalamus (which receives input from the neospinothalamic tract) projects to the primary somatosensory (SI) cortex, which is bordered anteriorly by the central sulcus. This arrangement is believed to provide the mechanism for the localization of pain.

The medial/intralaminar thalamic projections (after passage through limbic structures) extend to the second somatosensory cortex (SII), which lies on the inner face of the upper bank of the lateral sulcus (Treede et al, 2000). The role of SII is not well established, but may include the emotional and motivational aspects and the memory of pain.

Descending Pathways

People may not experience immediate pain, even though they are seriously injured. Physiologic mechanisms are involved, consistent with the closing of a physiologic 'gate' (Melzack and Wall, 1965). Neurones with cell bodies in periaqueductal grey matter and fibres in the dorsal column can inhibit the discharge of dorsal horn cells, thereby reducing nociceptive input. A feedback loop is formed, with input from the spinoreticular and palaeospinothalamic tracts, the reticular formation and the periaqueductal grey matter.

As pain is a warning system, it is uncertain why a mechanism for reducing nociception should exist. However, if you come across a sleeping lion in the jungle and step on a thorn as you back away, it is better that you continue to focus your attention on the lion, rather than scream and leap in the air. The pain-suppression pathway appears to be a component of a general sensory input regulation mechanism that allows us to ignore certain stimuli.

The ability of supraspinal components to reduce the experience of pain is consistent with the finding that relaxation and hypnosis (strong methods of focusing of attention) have well-established analgesic actions.

The physiologic 'gate' can also be closed at the segmental level, by activation of large neurones in the skin. This principle is well known to anyone who has grazed and rubbed their knee, and has found clinical utility in the application of heat and electrical currents to reduce pain.

References

Bonica J. *The Management of Pain*, 2nd edn. Lea & Febiger, Philadelphia, 1990a.

Bonica J. Anatomic and physiologic basis of nociception and pain. In: Bonica J (ed) *The Management of Pain*, 2nd edn. Lea & Febiger, Philadelphia, 1990b.

Brose W, Spiegel D. Neuropsychiatric aspects of pain management. In: Yudofsky S and Hales R (eds) *The American Psychiatric Textbook of Neuropsychiatry*, 2nd edn. American Psychiatric Press, Washington, DC, 1992: 245–75.

Haines D. *Fundamental Neuroscience*. Churchill Livingstone, New York, 1997.

Melzack R, Wall P. Pain mechanisms: a new theory. *Science* 1965; 150: 971–9.

Price D. Psychological and neural mechanisms of the affective dimensions of pain. *Science* 2000; 228: 1769–72.

Treede R, Apkarian A, Bromm B. Cortical representation of pain: functional characterization of nociceptive areas near the lateral sulcus. *Pain* 2000; 87: 113–17.

Wall P, Melzack R. *Textbook of Pain*. Churchill Livingstone, Edinburgh, 1999.

Woolf C, Mannion R. Neuropathic pain: aetiology, symptoms, mechanisms, and management. *Lancet* 1999; 353: 1959–64.

Plasticity and neuropathic pain

Acute pain is a warning signal that serves a necessary survival
function. Two types of acute pain can be recognized:
physiologic/normal pain and clinical (see Figure 4.1). In
physiologic/normal pain there is minimal or no tissue damage,
such as when one picks up, and quickly puts down, an
unexpectedly hot dinner plate (Woolf and Salter, 2000).

Clinical pain, on the other hand, is associated with severe
noxious insult and tissue damage. Two types can be
recognized: acute and chronic. Unlike acute pain, chronic
pain performs no useful function, representing instead a tragic
human burden. Three types of chronic pain can be
recognized: psychogenic, inflammatory and neuropathic.

Inflammation is a fundamental pathologic process, a
dynamic complex of cytologic and histologic reactions that
occur in affected blood vessels and adjacent tissues, in
response to an injury or abnormal stimulation, caused by a
physical, chemical or biologic agent. For present purposes,
inflammatory pain is most frequently associated with trauma

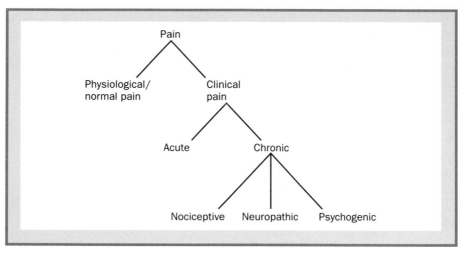

Figure 4.1
The pain tree, Physiological/normal pain is a distant relative of neuropathic pain and the other forms of chronic pain. There is, at most, a slight family resemblance.

and the 'inflammatory diseases'. An important recent finding is that neuropathic changes may be associated not only with direct trauma to neural tissue, but also with continuous or severe nociceptive input from inflammatory lesions (Terayama et al, 2000).

Neuropathic pain is defined as 'pain initiated or caused by a primary lesion or dysfunction in the nervous system' (Mersky and Bogduk, 1994). It may manifest very severe symptoms; it is usually chronic, always difficult to treat. It is poorly understood, and deserves special consideration. Neuropathic pain depends on neuroplasticity, that is, change in the function, chemistry and structure of neurones. Accordingly, it depends

on change in gene expression and phenotype (Hunt and Mantyh, 2001). For example, the biology of sensory neurones is maintained by growth factors for the innervated tissues, and following inflammation, changes in phenotype are triggered by changes in the factors released at the injury site.

The symptoms that suggest neuropathic pain include spontaneous pain, hyperalgesia and allodynia. The spontaneous pain is characteristically burning or shooting in nature. Hyperalgesia is an increased pain response to a suprathreshold noxious stimulus (that is, a painful stimulus hurts more than it should). Allodynia is the sensation of pain elicited by a non-noxious stimulus, such as the gentle touch of clothes or the bending of a cutaneous hair by a puff of wind. Spontaneous pain may be conceptualized as 'stimulus-independent' and hyperalgesia and allodynia as 'stimulus-dependent' pain.

Focusing on symptoms and aetiology has not provided a productive model for understanding or intervention. It has become clear that neuropathic pain does not have a single underlying mechanism. In fact an extensive range of mechanisms has been discovered. No particular injury or disease process is associated with a unique pain mechanism, and many different mechanisms may produce the same symptom. In any given patient suffering neuropathic pain, a number of mechanisms are usually operating at the same time, and they usually change over time.

The newly described neuropathic mechanisms operate at the peripheral, spinal cord and supraspinal levels (Taylor, 2001). We currently lack reliable methods of preventing the development of these mechanisms. We are unable to determine reliably, in the clinical setting, which particular mechanism/s is/are operating in a given patient. Finally, we lack a specific and effective therapeutic intervention for each mechanism. Understanding of these mechanisms, however, is growing, new interventions are being developed, and there is promise for the future. There is a basis for progress.

Even at this early stage, knowledge of the mechanisms is helpful to the clinician. It gives a better understanding of the mode of action of some of our rudimentary interventions. For example, in neuropathic pain the tricyclic antidepressants function not only on neurotransmitters but also as sodium channel blockers, thus reducing ectopic discharges (see below). Importantly, these mechanisms give a more complete understanding of the neuropathic pain patient. They give legitimacy to a range of claimed symptoms that have often been doubted by clinicians. They explain how pain can be felt when there is no activity and how activity may make pain worse. They explain how pain can be triggered by the slightest touch, how pain can spread beyond the site of trauma and, with the change of mechanisms over time, how one agent may be useful at one time but become frustratingly useless later on.

Predisposition

Trauma and inflammatory conditions are of aetiological importance, leading to local changes and subsequent phenotypic modification (Hunt and Mantyh, 2001). However, by no means all of those people exposed to trauma and inflammatory conditions develop neuropathic pain. There is now evidence of an inherited predisposition to chronic pain (Mogil et al, 1999).

There is evidence that a disturbed early life may result in brain changes and a predisposition to depression. Depression is common in chronic pain, and chronic pain is more common among the socially disadvantaged. Such threads have led to speculation that a disturbed early life may also predispose to chronic pain (Rome and Rome, 2000).

The mechanisms

Ectopic discharge

Spontaneous activity in normal primary sensory neurones is low. After injury, however, spontaneous ectopic discharges are observed in skeletal muscle afferents (Michaelis et al, 2000). These are the result of phenotypic changes in the nature of and distribution of sodium and calcium channels, which occur throughout the damaged neurone, including the dorsal root ganglion (DRG). These changes may not only result in spontaneous pain, but contribute to central sensitization (to be discussed below). Interestingly, after insult to a region, some uninjured neurones may also demonstrate ectopic discharge (Bridges et al, 2001).

Sensitization of sensory terminals

Nociceptor peripheral terminals of injured and uninjured neurones are sensitized by substance P, released from the terminals of local damaged neurones. Axons transmit potentials in both directions, and such agents are released by antidromic potentials, which proceed from ectopic discharges (Woolf and Mannion, 1999).

Cross-excitation

Injury may lead to disruption of glial sheaths. Adjacent denuded axons may make electrical or chemical contact, resulting in cross-excitation. Undamaged neurones may also become involved (Amir and Devor, 2000). When A-beta fibres activate C fibres, non-noxious stimuli may produce pain.

Neurotransmitter change

After injury, phenotypic change in the production of neurotransmitters of peripheral nerves may result in pain. A-beta fibres, which normally transmit non-noxious tactile messages, may begin to release pro-nociceptive transmitters, such as substance P, at the spinal cord (Noguchi et al, 1995). Thus, touch may cause pain.

Coupling between the sympathetic and sensory nervous systems

In normal physiologic conditions, the sympathetic nervous system cannot cause pain. Uninjured primary sensory nerve endings are not sensitive to catecholamines and are functionally distinct from the efferent sympathetic nervous system.

After injury, however, there are at least two mechanisms by which coupling between the sympathetic and sensory motor systems may be established, providing mechanisms for neuropathic pain. First, both injured and uninjured neurones develop alpha-adrenoreceptors, which makes them responsive to noradrenaline from sympathetic nerve terminals. (Injured neurones are also believed to be responsive to circulating adrenaline and noradrenaline.) Second, sprouting of sympathetic axons into the DRGs forms baskets around the cell bodies of sensory neurones and appears to be capable of causing depolarization (Woolf and Mannion, 1999).

In spite of these potential mechanisms, the actual proportion of cases of neuropathic pain in which there is significant contribution from the sympathetic nervous system is probably small. Current treatments of neuropathic pain that are aimed at the sympathetic system have produced equivocal results (Kingery, 1997).

Spinal cord reorganization

The normal arrangement is that primary afferent neurones terminate in particular layers of the dorsal horn of the spinal cord, synapsing with particular, predetermined second-order neurones. Lamina II receives nociceptor C-fibres exclusively. After nerve injury, however, there may be substantial degeneration and loss of the central terminals of C fibres in lamina II. There may be numbness. The central projections of surviving A-beta fibres in laminas III and IV may sprout into the territory vacated by the C-fibre terminals in lamina II and make contact with second-order pain transmission neurones (Woolf et al, 1995). Thus non-noxious information, such as proprioceptive information or touch, may be interpreted as being of noxious origin. This is a pathophysiological explanation for pain from movement and allodynia (Kohama et al, 2000).

Spinal cord increased excitability

Any prolonged or excessive sensory input from persistent inflammation or nerve injury may result in increased excitability in the spinal cord (Woolf and Wall, 1986). This has been called 'central sensitization'. Several mechanisms have been described. Nociceptor input may lead directly to sensitization of secondary dorsal horn neurones. Peripheral nerve injury may lead to elevated spinal dynorphin (endogenous opioid), which may sensitize the second-order neurones in the cord. Such elevation may be 'multisegmental', occurring at levels distant from the segment of the injured nerve, causing 'extraterritorial' neuropathic pain, or pain in a region not supplied by the damaged nerve (Malan et al, 2000).

With healing, central sensitization may

subside. However, through ectopic activity in A-beta neurones, it may be sustained indefinitely.

Spinal cord decreased inhibition

Nerve injury may result in death of inhibitory dorsal horn interneurones, which leads to disinhibition and the increased likelihood of dorsal horn neurones firing spontaneously or in an exaggerated manner (Woolf and Mannion, 1999). Decreased spinal cord gamma amino butyric acid (GABA) concentration and GABA receptor binding sites have been reported (Castro-Lopes et al, 1993). Thus the 'gate' can no longer be closed by stimulating intact peripheral A-beta fibres or via descending impulses from higher centres.

Supraspinal influences

The ability of descending fibres to inhibit nociception is well established. More recently, descending fibres with an ability to facilitate nociception have been reported. Evidence indicates that injury and persistent noxious input associated with inflammatory pain causes long-term changes in the activity of brain stem neurones that enhance facilitation and contribute to neuropathic pain (Ossipov et al, 2000). This facilitation appears to be driven by brain-stem cholecystokinin (Kovelowski et al, 2000).

The above findings are largely from single-cell neurophysiology studies of experimental animals. These techniques are not at present available in clinical practice. Valuable human information, however, can be derived from imaging and related studies.

The thalamus is believed to experience pain-related plastic change (Lenz et al, 2000). Quantitative sensory testing and neurophysiological and psychological examination of patients with complex regional pain syndrome suggest thalamic plasticity in chronic pain (Rommel et al, 2001). Regional blood flow changes have been observed in the basal ganglia of patients with chronic pain (Mountz et al, 1998). Altered facilitation and inhibition of the motor cortex using transcranial magnetic stimulation in two groups of patients with two painful disorders, fibromyalgia and rheumatoid arthritis, have been demonstrated by Salerno et al (2000). They hypothesized these findings were secondary to pain-induced changes in the basal ganglia.

Chronic back pain (Flor et al, 1997) and amputation (Wiech et al, 2000) are associated with spatial reorganization of somatosensory cortical mapping. Birbaumer et al (1995) have described 'corticalization' of chronic pain. Such changes have yet to be thoroughly investigated; however, it is probable that plastic brain changes secondary to pain are important in causing and maintaining neuropathic pain.

Treatment implications

Neuropathic pain is difficult to treat. We are waiting for the new understanding of the pathophysiologic mechanisms to lead the way. Clinical tests are required to identify which mechanisms are present, and new therapeutic options are also necessary to address each. Research is currently being conducted on many potentially useful pharmacological agents, including unique sodium channel blocker and nerve growth factors.

From the existing pain treatments, the non-steroidal anti-inflammatory drugs have little effect, and the use of opiates in neuropathic pain is a matter of debate (Rowbotham et al, 1998). Dorsal column stimulation and chronic epidural administration of a range of drugs using implanted devices are available at special centres. Woolf and Mannion (1999) described the former as controversial and the latter as not having been adequately assessed. Various anaesthetic blocks may provide temporary relief.

The tricyclic antidepressants and anticonvulsants have been the most useful agents over a number of decades. It has long been thought that the beneficial action of the tricyclics was related to increases in noradrenaline and serotonin in the dorsal horn. Recent evidence indicates that they reduce ectopic depolarization by a sodium channel blocking action. Carbamazepine has an established role in trigeminal neuralgia, and, along with sodium valproate, appears to have more general application in neuropathic pain. Gabapentin appears to have a place in the management of post-herpetic neuralgia and other neuropathies (Backonja et al, 1998). Lamotrigine and topiramate may prove to be useful.

In general, in chronic pain, it is important to recognize and treat concurrent depression and anxiety. This enables people to 'cope' with their pain and associated difficulties. Insomnia is common, can lead to dysphoria, and is usually responsive to tricyclics. Psychotherapy that focuses on cognitive behaviour may be of benefit. Patients are encouraged to take a logical and practical approach to their condition and life situation. They are encouraged to measure their self-worth using philosophical rather than physical productivity criteria. Meditation of various forms has a beneficial role, reducing anxiety and improving pain status (Kabat-Zinn et al, 1987). Compliance can be a problem, but this approach has high patient acceptance and has the advantage of being side-effect free, and strongly involves patients in their own care. Activity and independence is encouraged. While regular opioids are better avoided if possible, it is important not to leave patients with only psychological techniques when pain does crescendo. Tramadol or another suitable agent has a place as an 'as needed rescue package' when the activity recommended by the physician leads to an exacerbation of symptoms.

References

Amir R, Devor M. Functional cross-excitation between afferent A- and C-neurons in dorsal root ganglia. *Neuroscience* 2000; 95: 189–95.

Backonja M, Beydoun A, Edwards K, et al. Gabapentin for the symptomatic treatment of painful neuropathy in patients with diabetes mellitus: a randomized controlled trial. *Journal of the American Medical Association* 1998; 280: 1831–6.

Birbaumer N, Flor H, Lutzenberger W, Elbert T. Corticalization of chronic pain. In: Bromm B and Desmedt J (eds) *Pain and the Brain: From Nociception to Cognition. Advances in Pain Research and Therapy* Vol. 22. Raven Press, New York, 1995; 331–43.

Bridges D, Thompson S, Rice A. Mechanisms of neuropathic pain. *British Journal of Anaesthesia* 2001; 87: 12–26.

Castro-Lopes J, Tavares I, Coimbra A. GABA decreases in the spinal cord dorsal horn after peripheral neurectomy. *Brain Research* 1993; 620: 287–91.

Flor H, Christoph B, Elbert T, Birbaumer N. Extensive reorganization of primary somatosensory cortex in chronic back pain patients. *Neuroscience Letters* 1997; 224: 5–8.

Hunt S. Mantyh P. The molecular dynamics of pain control. *Neuroscience* 2001; 2: 83–91.

Kabat-Zinn J, Lipworth L, Burney R, Sellers W. Four-year follow-up of a meditation-based program for the self-regulation of chronic pain: treatment outcome and compliance. *Clinical Journal of Pain* 1987; 2: 159–73.

Kingery W. A critical review of controlled clinical trials for peripheral neuropathic pain and complex regional pain syndromes. *Pain* 1997; 73: 123–39.

Kohama I, Ishikawa K, Kocsis J. Synaptic reorganization in substantia gelatinosa after peripheral nerve neuroma fomation: aberrant innervation of lamina interneurons by A-beta afferents. *Journal of Neuroscience* 2000; 20: 1538–49.

Kovelowski C, Ossipov M, Sun H, Lai J, Malan T, Porreca F. Supraspinal cholecystokinin may drive tonic facilitation mechanisms to maintain neuropathic pain in the rat. *Pain* 2000; 87: 265–73.

Lenz F, Lee J, Garonzik I, Rowland L, Dougherty P, Hua S. Plasticity of pain-related neuronal activity in the human thalamus. *Progress in Brain Research* 2000; 129: 259–73.

Malan T, Ossipov M, Gardell L, Ibrahim M, Bian D, Lai J, Porreca F. Extraterritorial neuropathic pain correlates with multisegmental elevation of spinal dynorphin in nerve-injured rats. *Pain* 2000; 86: 185–94.

Mersky H, Bogduk N. *Classification of Chronic Pain*, 2nd edn. IASP Press, Seattle, 1994; 394.

Michaelis M, Liu X, Janig W. Axotomized and intact muscle afferents but not skin afferents develop ongoing discharges of dorsal root ganglion origin after peripheral nerve lesion. *Journal of Neuroscience* 2000; 20: 2742–8.

Mogil J, Wilson S, Bon K. Heritability of nociception II. 'Types' of nociception revealed by genetic correlation analysis. *Pain* 1999; 80: 83–93.

Mountz J, Bradley L, Alarcon G. Abnormal functional activity of the central nervous system in fibromyalgia syndrome. *American Journal of Medical Science* 1998; 315: 385–96.

Noguchi K, Kawai Y, Fukuoka T. Substance P induced by peripheral nerve injury in primary afferent sensory neurons and its effect on dorsal column nucleus neurons. *Journal of Neuroscience* 1995; 15: 7633–43.

Ossipov M, Lai J, Malan T, Porreca F. Spinal and supraspinal mechanisms of neuropathic pain. *Annals of New York Academy of Science* 2000; 909: 12–24.

Price D. Psychological and neural mechanisms of the affective dimension of pain. *Science* 2000; 288: 1769–72.

Rome H, Rome J. Limbically augmented pain syndrome (LAPS): kindling, corticolimbic sensitization, and the convergence of affective and sensory symptoms in chronic pain disorder. *Pain Medicine* 2000; 1: 7–23.

Rommel O, Malin J, Zenz M, Janig W. Quantitative sensory testing, neurophysiological and psychological examination in patients with complex regional pain syndrome and hemisensory deficits. *Pain* 2001; 93: 279–93.

Rowbotham M, Kalso E, McQuay H, Wiesenfeld-Hallin Z (eds) *The Debate over Opioids and Neuropathic Pain. Opioid Sensitivity of Chronic Non-cancer Pain.* IASP Press, Seattle, 1998; 218: 307–17.

Salerno A, Thomas E, Olive P, Blotman F, Picot M, Georgesco M. Motor cortical dysfunction disclosed by single and double magnetic stimulation in patients with fibromyalgia. *Clinical Neurophysiology* 2000; 111: 994–1001.

Taylor B. Pathophysiologic mechanisms of neuropathic pain. *Current Pain and Headache Reports* 2001; 5: 151–61.

Terayama R, Guan Y, Dubner R, Ren K. Activity-induced plasticity in brain stem pain modulatory circuits after inflammation. *Neuroreport* 2000; 11: 1915–19.

Wiech K, Preissl H, Birbaumer N. Neuroimaging of chronic pain: phantom limb and musculoskeletal pain. *Scandinavian Journal of Rheumatology* 2000; 29: 13–18.

Woolf C, Wall P. Relative effectiveness of C primary afferent fibers of different origins in evoking a prolonged facilitation of the flexor reflex in the rat. *Journal of Neuroscience* 1986; 6: 1433–42.

Woolf C, Shortland P, Reynolds M, Riding J, Doubell T, Coggeshall R. Reorganization of central terminals of myelinated primary afferents in the rat dorsal horn following peripheral axotomy. *Journal of Comparative Neurology* 1995; 360: 121–34.

Woolf C, Mannion R. Neuropathic pain: aetiology, symptoms, mechanisms, and management. *Lancet* 1999; 353: 1959–64.

Woolf C, Salter M. Neuronal plasticity: increasing the gain in pain. *Science* 2000; 288: 1765–8.

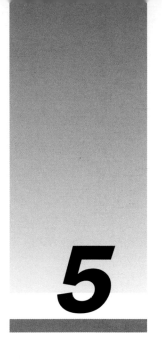

The biopsychosocial model in chronic pain

5

'A biopsychosocial model . . . includes the patient as well as the illness . . .'

George L Engel 1977

Before focusing on the biopsychosocial model, it is worth considering two less satisfactory models.

Biomedical model

The biomedical model conceptualizes disorders as arising from physical causes. It looks to eradicate such causes with the expectation that the resolution of the disorders and a return to normal function will automatically follow.

This model is well suited to the treatment of certain infections and fractures. It is less well suited to the management of mental illness.

The biomedical model is suited to the management of acute pain where a close relationship usually exists between the symptom and the degree of tissue injury. Narrow focus, however, renders the biomedical model unsatisfactory in chronic pain. Slavish devotion to the biomedical model in chronic pain, with progression to repeated invasive techniques, is unlikely to be beneficial and may end in iatrogenic complications.

Operant model

This model of chronic pain has roots in learning theory (Fordyce, 1976). For a critical review see Roth (2000). The observations were made that pain is communicated by 'pain behaviours' and that chronic pain persists beyond the expected healing time. This led to the theory that while acute pain was associated with appropriate acute pain behaviour, chronic pain behaviour was reinforced or maintained by environmental factors. In operant theory, chronic pain behaviours are maintained by financial rewards, the attention of others and the avoidance of duty. Pain behaviour rather than pain experience became the focus of clinical attention. It is unclear whether proponents believe that chronic patients are suffering pain and whether or not changing behaviour reduces any such suffering.

The operant pain model was enthusiastically embraced. It became and remains, a central plank of some intensive multidisciplinary treatment programmes, supported by cognitive therapy, occupational therapy, physiotherapy and medication reduction.

However, theoretical objections have been raised. Lacy (1985) pointed out that operant behaviours should result in predictable results,

but that this was not the case with chronic pain behaviour, as some environmental figures provided support while others withdrew from the patient. Jaynes (1985) pointed out that the reinforcer/rewards should have the same effect on every patient, but that does not hold in the chronic pain scenario either, as some patients find money positively rewarding, while others are relatively indifferent. Roth (2000) points out that some losses that are generally regarded as among the unwanted consequences of chronic pain, such as the loss of work status, are regarded as gains in operant pain theory.

While some pain behaviours communicate that the patient is experiencing pain, this does not necessarily imply that such behaviour is under conscious control. There is strong evidence that facial pain behaviour has an evolutionary (survival) basis and that much of it is involuntary in origin (Williams, unpublished). It is possible to exert some control over the pain behaviour of facial expression, but it cannot be completely hidden and is detectable by observers (Poole and Craig, 1992). There is evidence that patients may openly demonstrate pain behaviour when in the presence of supportive and caring people (Block et al, 1980). But this may be interpreted in many ways. Williams (unpublished) offers a credible interpretation, proposing that when suffering patients are in the presence of supportive people they are able to release the control they have been exerting over their pain behaviour, which may lead to an apparent but not an actual exaggeration. An analogy is drawn with grieving: the 'brave' individual is able to remain composed until a supportive or 'safe' individual expresses sympathy.

While some chronic pain patients are undoubtedly motivated by secondary gains, operant pain theory cannot be accepted as a generalized explanation of chronic pain (Schmidt, 1987).

Biopsychosocial model

The biopsychosocial model of illness (Engel, 1977) highlights the importance of biological/medical, psychological/psychiatric and social/environmental contributions to aetiology and therapy. It is a guiding concept in psychiatry and comprehensive family medicine.

The biopsychosocial model is a useful concept in pain medicine and is consistent with the International Association for the Study of Pain definition: 'Pain is an unpleasant sensory and emotional experience associated with actual or potential tissue damage, or described in terms of such damage' (Merskey, 1979).

Rome and Rome (2000) have proposed a structural process for the biopsychosocial model of chronic pain. They reviewed information suggesting that disturbing early life experiences lead to plastic brain changes

that predispose the individual to depression in adult life. They speculate that these changes also predispose the individual to chronic pain, as sensitization of similar corticolimbic structures could be involved. This theory might help to explain the high prevalence of comorbidity of chronic pain and psychiatric disorders and the pain-prone disorders that are discussed below.

The biological/medical component

The biological/medical or physical basis of pain is not contested. The chapters on Anatomy and physiology, Plasticity and neuropathic pain, and Pharmacotherapy give relevant information on aetiology and therapy.

Other physical/medical forms of pain therapy include trigger point injection, temporary neural blockade, chemical and radiofrequency neurolysis, cordotomy, massage, acupuncture, intraspinal drug administration, transcutaneous electrical nerve stimulation (TENS), dorsal column stimulation and deep brain stimulation.

The psychological/psychiatric component

The contention of the International Association for the Study of Pain that pain involves 'emotional experience' raises the question of mechanism. In exploring this issue some material is presented here that could also have been listed under the above heading of 'The biological/medical component' – this testifies to the unity of mind and body.

Darwin (1872) conceptualized emotion as having evolutionary significance, as being a mechanism that facilitates communication and behaviour, and thereby, survival of the individual and the species. Later, Papez (1937) described the limbic brain as 'the hypothalamus, the anterior thalamic nuclei, the gyrus cinguli, the hippocampus and their connections' and proposed it as 'a harmonious mechanism which may elaborate the functions of central emotion'. These observations were elaborated by MacLean (1952, 1990) who emphasized the importance of the limbic system and its functions to evolution.

Communication between the periphery and the brain was reviewed by Chapman (1995). He found that, in the nervous system, the differentiation between sensory and emotional processing begins at the dorsal horn of the spinal cord. Information serving the sensory experience proceeds via the spinothalamic pathways and that serving the emotional experience proceeds via the spinoreticular pathways. With respect to emotion, important among the reticular formation projections is the dorsal noradrenergic bundle (DNB), which originates in the pontine locus coeruleus (LC) and passes upward in the median forebrain bundle (MFB) to project throughout the limbic brain and the neocortex.

Neurones from the medullary region of the reticular formation form the ventral noradrenergic bundle (VNB), which also passes upwards in the MFB, projects to the hypothalamus, and provides the neurophysiological link between tissue injury and the endocrine system. Hypothalamic activity releases cortisol, which has wide-ranging effects on the brain, including modification of the firing rate of the limbic forebrain. Also, the hypothalamus has neural links with the limbic brain and the autonomic nervous system.

Melzack (1999) has emphasized the importance of the interconnections between the endocrine, autonomic and limbic systems, which, in addition to the neural and endocrine factors, include the endogenous opioids.

The immune system is another mechanism by which tissue damage results in limbic brain activation. Within seconds of tissue damage, cytokines are released from blood cells. They immediately cross the blood–brain barrier and stimulate the hypothalamus, and thus the adrenal medulla and the limbic system. The cytokine interleukin-1 stimulates the hypothalamus to produce fever. Dantzer and Kelley (1989) report that increased cytokine release results in malaise, fatigue, sleepiness, anorexia, apathy and irritability. Experimental immune activation using an endotoxin produced negative emotional states and decreased performance in memory function tests (Reichenberg et al, 2001). These effects were considered to be due to cytokine release, and this study has relevance to a range of clinical conditions, including infectious and autoimmune diseases (including multiple sclerosis), cardiac disease, brain trauma and neuro-degenerative diseases.

Psychological factors in aetiology

Common sense and clinical experience both suggest that the mental state can impact on pain. Most forms of mental distress result in increased muscle tension, which leads to increased pain. (Mental distress, here, includes normal emotional arousal as well as the diagnosable conditions of anxiety and depression. It also includes other mental disorders in which emotional arousal may be a feature, such as schizophrenia.)

The physiology of increased muscle tension leading to increased pain has not been definitively elucidated. Contributing factors, however, include an increased mechanoreceptor inflow, increased mechanical forces applied to nociceptor endings and increased local metabolites with the potential to sensitize nociceptor endings.

Pain also leads to increased muscle tension by various mechanisms. It triggers the autonomic fight or flight reaction, in which increased muscle tension prepares the organism to respond to threat with quick strong movements. Also, an automatic

'splinting' or tightening of muscles occurs to reduce the movement of painful structures.

Thus, positive feedback loops develop, in which pain leads to emotional tension or splinting, which lead to further pain.

It is also a common experience that pain is experienced as more intense at night. While a circadian explanation could be involved, an important feature is the reduction of stimuli. Other people are asleep and unavailable, and the television offers little of interest. There is thus no distraction, and pain that prevents sleep becomes the focus of attention.

'Worry' or apprehension, concern and anticipation of future adverse events or misfortunes are a very common human problem. They form a feature of generalized anxiety disorder, but are also present to a lesser extent in a much broader section of the population. Such worries may focus on external possibilities, such as floods or loss of spouse or job, or on internal events such as loss of beauty or virility or onset of disease. Worry is unpleasant, and often uncontrollable. A frequent accompanying feature is muscle tension. Thus what can be called 'normal' worrying may accentuate muscle tension and pain. Worry is even more likely and potent when there is 'something to worry about', that is, when disease or injury has brought loss or potential loss of income or family, or the prospect of long-term health problems. Finally, particular difficulties can be anticipated when the worrying of the past has focused on concerns about disease or disability.

Various formal psychological theories have been offered as explanation for medically inexplicable pain. Freud (1953 [1893]) described hysteria as the transformation of unacceptable unconscious conflicts into bodily pain as a means of preventing conscious awareness. In his seminal and sensitive paper, 'Psychogenic pain and the pain-prone patient', Engel (1959) emphasized the importance of guilt in the generation of chronic pain. Blumer and Heilbronn (1982) argued that chronic pain is a variant of depressive disorder or 'masked depression'. They introduced the term 'pain-prone disorder' in which hard-working people with limited capacity to express emotions (alexithymia), after loss or disappointment, with or without painful injury or ailment, become dependent and anergic and suffer continuous pain. All these psychological explanations probably explain the symptoms of occasional chronic pain patients, but not the majority.

In a large prospective study of the onset of forearm pain (Macfarlane et al, 2000), mechanical and psychological factors were identified. The important mechanical factors were repetitive movements of the hand and wrist. The most important psychological factor was dissatisfaction with support from colleagues or supervisors. The authors cautioned against terms such as 'repetitive strain injury' because they imply a single uniform aetiology and neglect major psychosocial contributions.

There is a high prevalence of psychiatric disorder among those with chronic pain disorder (see the chapter on Pain and psychiatric comorbidity). One disorder may exacerbate the other: hence psychiatric disorders need to be considered in the aetiology and treatment of chronic pain.

Psychological factors in treatments

The psychological support provided by clinical staff and family and friends is important in maintaining a positive attitude and encouraging efforts to regain function. Where psychological contributions are particularly important, psychological treatments such as dynamic psychotherapy or cognitive behaviour therapy have an important place. Psychotherapy also has a place where biological contributions are of primary importance, but adjustment to changed circumstances is proving difficult.

The pain-management 'system' and the less than optimal current treatments are a cause of great frustration and anger (Walker et al, 1999). While these emotions may not have initiated the pain, they play an important role in perpetuating distress. It is important to treat patients with respect and without unnecessary delay. It is best to keep them informed and involved as a means of helping them to deal with demoralization and anger.

Social/environmental/cultural component

- Disease: biological or pathological changes that one 'has'.
- Illness: psychological or the way one 'feels' when diseased.
- Sick: one acts or behaves the role 'given' by society.

In sociological terms there are distinctions between illness, disease and sickness. Illness is the subjective sense that one is not well. Disease is an objective pathology of the body such as cancer. Sickness is the condition of those who are socially recognized as unwell. To put this in another way, illness is a 'psychological' phenomenon in that one 'feels' ill, disease is a 'biological' phenomenon in that one 'has' a disease and sickness is a 'social' phenomenon in that one 'acts or behaves' in the manner of a sick person (Twaddle and Hessler, 1986). Difficulties may arise when an individual has one or two of these without the third. An individual with cancer and obvious signs of the disease may refuse to accept the sick role, including consulting a doctor. A more common disjunction is when an individual claims the sick role but others do not accept that there is disease. The term 'abnormal illness behaviour' can be applied in both of these examples.

Cultural factors are also important in the expression of illness and the granting of the sick role. Considerable ethnic differences can be found between groups living in the same country. Zborowski (1969) looked at whites living in the USA. Italo-Americans were very 'present-orientated' about pain and were primarily concerned about obtaining immediate relief. Jews were more 'future-orientated' and more concerned about the long-term meaning of pain. Anglo-Saxons complained less and took a more detached, 'unemotional' view of symptoms.

Asians living in Britain are twice as likely, in comparison to Europeans, to consult their general practitioner (Balarajan et al, 1989), and musculoskeletal pain is one of the most common reasons for consultation (OPCS, 1995). Non-specific musculoskeletal pain, low back pain and soft-tissue conditions are more common in Pakistanis living in England than in those living in Pakistan (Hameed and Gibson, 1997). However, Pakistanis required less postoperative analgesia than European patients, although pain scores were observed to be similar (Houghton et al, 1992). Research indicates that Asians living in Britain are significantly disadvantaged, and this may be reflected in the difference in pain complaints.

Cultural values and the potency of stigma influence whether the distress is perceived and reported in psychological or in somatic terms (Raguram et al, 1996). Depressed Chinese patients most commonly present to general practitioners with complaints of somatic symptoms, including pain (Cheung et al, 1981). Ware and Kleinman (1992) compared Chinese suffering neurasthenia and North Americans suffering chronic fatigue syndrome. They argued that 'pain and suffering in society are manifested in pain and suffering in the body'. They supported the claim that somatic symptoms form part of a 'hidden transcript', a covert unofficial discourse that takes place out of sight of the wielders of power, and a way of addressing the desire for change in social life.

The operant model of pain has been described above under a dedicated heading. It is built on learning theory, and could be listed with psychological contributions; however, the purported rewards are derived from the social environment, and include the promise of money, the attention of others and the avoidance of duty. These so-called rewards cannot be universally applied, however: for example, while some may find the avoidance of duty to be a positive, just as many others find loss of social role to be a strong negative aspect of chronic pain. An alternative explanation has been offered for the apparent exaggeration of pain behaviour when patients suffering chronic pain are in the company of supportive people. Williams (unpublished) has proposed that in the company of supportive people, patients suffering chronic pain are able to release their suppression of, or stop hiding, their pain behaviour. There is evidence that pain behaviour has evolutionary origins and that animals are 'hard-wired' to elicit care that may promote survival.

Nevertheless, common sense and clinical experience suggest that a patient whose pain behaviour elicits excessive attention and protection from the social environment will often be slower to move out of this role than a patient whose social environment is less attentive and protective. Optimally, a balance is found when the patient feels valued and supported but also encouraged to strive for independence.

Group activities as well as group therapy have a place, providing for ventilation and inspiration through association with similarly afflicted peers.

References

Balarajan R, Yuen P, Soni Raleigh V. Ethnic differences in general practitioner consultations. *British Journal of Medicine* 1989; 299: 958–60.

Block A, Kremer E, Gaylor M. Behavioral treatment of chronic pain: the spouse as a discriminative cue for pain behavior. *Pain* 1980; 9: 243–52.

Blumer D, Heilbronn M. Chronic pain as a variant of depressive disease. The pain prone disorder. *Journal of Nervous and Mental Disorders* 1982; 170: 381–406.

Chapman C. The affective dimension of pain: a model. In: Bromm B, Desmedt J (eds) *Pain and the Brain: From Nociception to Cognition, Advances in Pain Research and Therapy* Vol. 22. Raven Press Ltd, New York, 1995; 283–301.

Cheung F, Lau B, Waldmann E. Somatization among Chinese depressives in general practice. *International Journal of Psychiatry Medicine* 1981; 10: 361–74.

Dantzer R, Kelley K. Stress and immunity: an integrated view of relationships between the brain and the immune system. *Life Sciences* 1989; 44: 1995–2008.

Darwin C. *The Expression of the Emotions in Man and Animals.* John Murray, London, 1872.

Engel G. 'Psychogenic' pain and the pain-prone patient. *American Journal of Medicine* 1959; 26: 899–918.

Engel G. The need for a new medical model: a challenge for biomedicine. *Science* 1977; 196: 129–36.

Fordyce W. *Behavioral Methods for Chronic Pain and Illness.* Mosby, St Louis, MO, 1976.

Freud S. On the psychical mechanisms of hysterical phenomena. *The Standard Edition of the Complete Psychological Works of Sigmund Freud,* Volume 3 (1893) Edited and translated by James Strachey. Hogarth Press, London, 1953; 25–42.

Hameed K, Gibson T. A comparison of the prevalence of rheumatoid arthritis and other rheumatic diseases amongst Pakistanis living in England and Pakistan. *British Journal of Rheumatology* 1997; 36: 781–5.

Houghton I, Aun C, Lau J. Inter-ethnic differences in postoperative pethidine requirements. *Anaesthesia and Intensive Care* 1992; 20: 52–5.

Jaynes J. Sensory pain and conscious pain. *Behavior and Brain Science* 1985; 8: 61–3

Kleinman A. Culture and somatic experience: the social course of illness in neurasthenia and chronic fatigue syndrome. *Psychosomatic Medicine* 1992; 54: 546–60.

Lacy H. Pain behavior: how to define this operant. *Behavior and Brain Science* 1985; 8: 64–5.

Macfarlane G, Hunt I, Silman A. Role of mechanical and psychosocial factors in the onset of forearm pain: prospective population base study. *British Medical Journal* 2000; 321: 676–9.

MacLean P. Some psychiatric implications of physiological studies on frontotemporal portions of the limbic system (visceral brain). *Electroencephalography and Clinical Neurophysiology* 1952; 4: 407–18.

MacLean P. *The Triune Brain in Evolution: Role in Paleocerebral Functions.* Plenum Press, New York, 1990.

Melzack R. Pain and stress: a new perspective. In: Gatchel R, Turk D (eds) *Psychosocial Factors in Pain.* The Guilford Press, New York, 1999; 89–106.

Merskey H. Pain terms: a list with definitions and notes on usage. Recommended by the International Association for the Study of Pain (IASP) Subcommittee on Taxonomy. Pain 1979; 6: 249–52.

OPCS (Office of Population Census and Surveys), The Royal College of General Practitioners, Department of Health and Social Security. *Morbidity Statistics from General Practice: Fourth National Study 1991–1992.* HMSO, London, 1995.

Papez J. A proposed mechanism of emotion. *Archives of Neurology and Psychiatry* 1937; 38: 723–43.

Poole G, Craig K. Judgements of genuine, suppressed and faked facial expressions of pain. *Journal of Personality and Social Psychology* 1992; 63: 797–805.

Raguram R, Weiss M, Channabasavanna S, Devins G. Stigma, depression and somatization in South India. *American Journal of Psychiatry* 1996; 15: 1043–9.

Reichenberg A, Yirmiya R, Schuld A, Kraus T, Haack M, Morag A, Pollmacher T. Cytokine-associated emotional and cognitive disturbances in humans. *Archives of General Psychiatry* 2001; 58: 445–52.

Rome H, Rome J. Limbically augmented pain syndrome (LAPS): kindling, corticolimbic sensitization, and the convergence of affective and sensory symptoms in chronic pain disorder. *Pain Medicine* 2000; 1: 7–23.

Roth R. Psychogenic models of chronic pain: a selective review and critique. In: Massie MJ (ed) *Pain: What Psychiatrists Need to Know.* (Review of Psychiatry Series, Vol. 19, No 2, Washington, DC, Oldham J and Riba M, series eds). American Psychiatric Press, 2000; 89–131.

Schmidt A. The behavioral management of pain: a criticism of a response. *Pain* 1987; 30: 285–91.

Twaddle A, Hessler R. *A Sociology of Health,* 2nd edn. Macmillan, New York, 1986.

Walker J, Holloway I, Sofaer B. In the system: the lived experience of chronic back pain from the perspectives of those seeking help from pain clinics. *Pain* 1999; 80: 621–8.

Ware N, Kleinman A. Culture and somatic experience: the social course of illness in neurasthenia and chronic fatigue syndrome. *Psychosomatic Medicine* 1992; 54: 546–60.

Williams A. Facial expression of pain: an evolutionary account (unpublished manuscript).

Zborowski M. *People in Pain.* Jossey-Bass, San Francisco, 1969.

Biopsychosocial pain and diagnostic systems

6

'The task of the real intellectual consists of analyzing illusions in order to discover their causes.'

Arthur Miller

The biopsychosocial model draws attention to the biological/physical, psychological/psychiatric and social/environmental contributions to disorders, diseases and conditions. It was described over two decades ago and is well regarded. It is a useful model when considering chronic pain. This chapter examines the major diagnostic systems for evidence of elements of the biopsychosocial model.

Current taxonomy has been criticized for failing to identify the multifactorial nature of pain, and an alternative, sign–symptom-based approach is recommended (Nicholson, 2000). Any such approach would be enriched by including psychosocial signs and symptoms.

Classification of Chronic Pain

Classification of Chronic Pain (Merskey and Bogduk, 1994) is the work of the Task Force on Taxonomy of the International Association for the Study of Pain. It was developed because pain was not comprehensively classified by the other taxonomies. This system incorporates all forms of chronic pain and codes according to five axes.

Axis I records the site of the pain. This is relatively straightforward. Example categories are head, face and mouth, cervical region and upper shoulders and upper limbs.

Axis II records the system that is involved. Systems such as the gastrointestinal and genitourinary systems have a single category each. The nervous system has two categories, one for the presence of a physical disturbance or dysfunction and the other for psychological, psychiatric and social conditions.

Axis III records the temporal characteristics and the pattern of occurrence of the pain. Examples of options include single episode, recurring regularly and recurring irregularly.

Axis IV records the patient statement of intensity and the time since onset. The intensity is recorded as mild, moderate or severe. The duration options are less than one month, one month to six months and greater than six months.

Axis V records aetiology. There are relatively straightforward categories such as neoplasm. There are two categories that involve psychological issues. One, called 'dysfunctional', includes pains with a psychophysiological basis. Examples include tension headache, which may or may not be a symptom of an anxiety disorder. The other is called 'psychological origin', and examples include 'conversion hysteria' and 'depressive hallucinations'.

Classification of Chronic Pain is a valuable contribution to the field of pain medicine. The psychological/psychiatric and social/environmental contributions receive some attention. Axis II is designed to code the relevant system, and has two categories for the nervous system, depending on whether there is a physical disturbance or dysfunction, or a psychological, psychiatric or social problem. Thus this axis, which deals with systems, is in danger of being confounded by aetiological factors. Further, Axis V, which is designed to code for aetiology, has a category called 'dysfunctional' that may have an anxiety disorder as a root cause, and another category called 'psychological origin' that may have 'conversion hysteria' as a root cause (a condition that may result from an anxiety-provoking situation such as warfare). Thus pain with similar psychological/psychiatric contributions may be placed in different aetiological categories. Finally, in the 'psychological origin' category, of the two examples given, one is a psychiatric disorder (conversion hysteria) and the other is a psychiatric symptom (depressive hallucination). Thus, the psychological/psychiatric and social/cultural contributions are superficially and confusingly presented.

Classification of Chronic pain elegantly and comprehensively classifies chronic pain from the biological/medical perspective. The International Association for the Study of Pain appears to be sympathetic to the biopsychosocial model. The fact that the psychological/psychiatric and social/environmental contributions to chronic pain are not more clearly reflected in Classification of Chronic Pain is testimony to the difficulty of this task.

International Classification of Disease – Version 10 (ICD-10)

ICD-10 (World Health Organization, 1992) is a comprehensive system that deals with the full spectrum of human diseases and extends over many volumes. It relies heavily on the biological/medical contributions, using combinations of system and aetiology in the classificatory process. It provides for psychological contributions to pain in the following ways.

'Histrionic elaboration of organically caused pain' is mentioned. Such behaviour is recognized in clinical practice. (Contrary to the thinking of some, statements to this effect can be made while fully respecting the dignity of the patient.)

'Psychological and behavioural factors associated with disorders or diseases classified elsewhere' is a useful category. 'Classified elsewhere' refers to classification elsewhere in the system, based on physical/medical criteria. Tension headache is an example. Mental tension may lead to muscular tension that in turn leads to headache. If the diagnostic criteria for a mental disorder are satisfied, that diagnosis is also recorded.

Persistent somatoform pain disorder is described as 'severe, and distressing pain, which cannot be explained fully by a physiological process or a physiological disorder. Pain occurs in association with emotional conflict or psychological problems that are sufficient to allow the conclusion that they are the main causative influences.' In practice it is often difficult to elaborate fully the predicted 'emotional conflict or psychological problems'. Patients may not have full insight into such issues, and may angrily deny the possibility of important psychological factors. Older classifications of 'hysteria' (Freud, 1953 [1893]) and the more recent dynamically orientated 'pain-prone personality disorder' (Engel, 1959) would be here incorporated.

Pain can be experienced during the course of depressive disorder, being placed under the heading of 'other depressive episodes', which incorporates the older diagnoses of atypical and masked depression. This is consistent with the work of Blumer and Heilbronn (1982). Theoretically, pain could present as a hallucination or delusion in psychotic depression; but in practice this is extremely rare.

Pain can be experienced as a hallucinatory phenomenon during the course of schizophrenia. However, in such cases other symptoms will be present on examination and the diagnosis should not be difficult.

The ICD-10 alerts to the possibility that reports of pain may be exaggerated (histrionic elaboration) and recognizes that psychological factors may exacerbate organically caused pain to cause what has been classified as a painful organic disorder ('psychological and behavioural factors associated with disorders or diseases elsewhere classified'). It also describes pain arising from psychiatric disorders (persistent somatoform pain disorder, depression and schizophrenia).

The ICD-10 is predominantly a biological/medical classificatory system. As has been detailed in the above paragraph, there is some effort to credit the importance of psychological contributions. There is mention of the use of 'a culturally acceptable explanation' under the heading of 'somatoform disorders', but this is exceptional. While a most useful diagnostic system, the ICD-10 does not fully incorporate the biopsychosocial model.

Diagnostic and Statistical Manual, 4th Edition (DSM-IV)

The DSM-IV (American Psychiatric Association, 1994) is concerned with mental disorders. It is a multiaxial (five axes) system.

Axis I records the main mental diagnoses (one or more), except Personality Disorder and Mental Retardation.

Axis II records Personality Disorders and Mental Retardation. It may also be used to list maladaptive personality features and defensive mechanisms. The listing of Personality Disorder and Mental Retardation on a separate axis ensures that these important aspects receive attention.

Axis III records any General Medical Conditions. These are coded according to ICD-9CM.

Axis IV reports Psychosocial and Environmental Problems that may affect the diagnosis, treatment and prognosis. Included here are negative life events, familial or other interpersonal stresses, and inadequacy of social support.

Axis V is the patient's Global Assessment of Functioning. It is useful in determining the impact of the condition, in planning treatment and in predicting outcome.

An Axis I diagnosis of Pain Disorder requires the satisfaction of five criteria. Important features are that pain is the predominant focus of clinical attention, that it causes significant distress and impairment and that psychological factors are judged to have an important role in the onset, severity, exacerbation, or maintenance of the pain.

Two subtypes are available: (1) Pain Disorder Associated With Psychological Factors (here psychological factors are judged to have a major role) and (2) Pain Disorder Associated With Both Psychological Factors and General Medical Condition.

Pain disorder associated with a general medical condition is not considered to be a mental disorder and is placed on Axis III.

The DSM-IV, through the multiaxial arrangement, approximates to the biopsychosocial model. Axis I records whether psychological factors play the major or an ancillary role. Axis II also calls for attention to be paid to psychological factors. Axis III records potentially contributing biological factors. Axis IV takes special account of the psychosocial and environmental problems, while Axis V takes account of the impact on the ability to function, which will determine the response of the environment.

Summary

Elements of the biopsychosocial model have been incorporated into Classification of Chronic Pain, ICD-10 and DSM-IV. The last of these systems appears to contain more such features than the other two systems.

References

American Psychiatric Association. *Diagnostic and Statistical Manual of Mental Disorders*, 4th edn. American Psychiatric Association, Washington, DC, 1994.

Blumer D, Heilbronn M. Chronic pain as a variant of depressive disease: the pain prone disorder. *Journal of Nervous and Mental Disease* 1982; 170: 381–406.

Engel G. 'Psychogenic' pain and the pain-prone patient. *American Journal of Medicine* 1959; 26: 899–918.

Freud S. On the psychical mechanisms of hysterical phenomena. In: *The Standard Edition of the Complete Psychological Works of Sigmund Freud*, Vol 3 Edited and translated by James Strachey. Hogarth Press, London, 1953 [1893]; 25–42.

Merskey H, Bogduk N. *Classification of Chronic Pain*. 2nd edn. IASP Press, Seattle, 1994.

Nicholson B. Taxonomy of pain. *Clinical Journal of Pain* 2000; 16: S114-17.

World Health Organization. *The ICD-10 Classification of Mental and Behavioural Disorders Clinical Descriptions and Diagnostic Guidelines*. World Health Organization, Geneva, 1992.

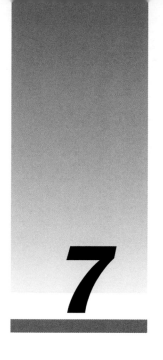

Pain and psychiatric comorbidity

7

'It has been proven that cigarettes are a major cause of statistics.'

Anonymous

It is important to emphasize the high prevalence of psychiatric disorder among patients with chronic pain. Evidence suggests that, in some cases, chronic pain leads to psychiatric disorder (Fishbain et al, 1997), while in other cases, psychiatric disorder leads to pain (Blumer and Heilbronn, 1982). Each of these pathways is right for different patients (Dworkin and Gitlin, 1991). In some cases this concurrence must be coincidental.

In a wide range of disorders, from diabetes to cancer, the treatment of concomitant psychiatric disorders contributes to a better clinical outcome. While randomized double blind trials have not been conducted to test the practice, common sense and clinical wisdom support the treatment of psychiatric disorders when they coexist with chronic pain (Atkinson et al, 1986; Dworkin and Gitlin, 1991; Sullivan et al, 1992; Fishbain, 1999), irrespective of the supposed precedence. At best, concomitant psychiatric disorders will delay recovery and increase suffering; at worst, they will contribute to death by suicide.

Psychiatric disorders overall

- Depression – probably >30%
- Anxiety – probably >40%
- Personality disorder – probably >50%.

Atkinson et al (1986) used Research Diagnostic Criteria in their study of 52 patients admitted to a neurosurgery unit for the treatment of pain, and found 78.4% to be suffering from a mental disorder. Merskey et al (1987) used self-assessment questionnaires in their study of 378 patients from four different pain services. Using the General Health Questionnaire, they found possible mental illness in 65.3% and probable mental illness in 41% of patients. These are different studies, as Atkinson et al (1986) considered inpatients and Merskey et al (1987) considered outpatients. However, even if the lower figures of Merskey et al (1987) are accepted, the concurrence is high, making psychiatric assessment and treatment in chronic pain an important contribution.

Depression

Depression is the psychiatric disorder that has received the most attention, and is present in those with chronic pain in the range 10%–100%.

Pilowsky et al (1977) examined 100 patients attending a pain clinic using the Levine–Pilowsky Depression Questionnaire.

They found 10% suffered an unequivocal depressive syndrome (endogenous-psychotic depression or reactive-neurotic depression). This finding was less than half that for the next lowest assessment. The Levine–Pilowsky Depression Questionnaire has not been used in subsequent studies of pain populations, and may not be suited to the task.

Blumer and Heilbronn (1982) coined the term 'pain-prone disorder' and conceptualize chronic pain as a variant of depression and thus, by definition, considered all those suffering chronic pain to be suffering depression. While this work drew attention back to the importance of psychological factors in chronic pain, the hypothesis that all chronic pain resulted from depression in individuals with psychodynamic vulnerability was not accepted (Turk and Flor, 1984).

Davidson et al (1985) examined 57 patients with chronic pain using the Research Diagnostic Criteria and found major depression in 42% and minor depression in 37%, for a total with depressive disorder of 79%. Atkinson et al (1986) examined 52 patients with chronic pain using the Research Diagnostic Criteria and found major depression in 21.6% and minor depression in 44.2%, for a total with depressive disorder of 65.8%.

Sullivan et al (1992) reviewed the studies of depression in chronic low back pain and concluded that the levels of depression were approximately four times greater than that reported in the general population. Probably, one-third of those with a range of chronic pain suffer major depression Roth (2000).

Anxiety

Fear is akin to anxiety, and differentiation is often difficult. Fear/anxiety is a response to threat and is ubiquitous in acute pain. In chronic pain it is less common, but nevertheless frequently present. Wise and Taylor (1990) confirm that anxiety is commonly associated with most chronic medical conditions. As has been mentioned, depression is frequently present and anxiety symptoms are common in depression.

By contrast with depression, no theory has been advanced that chronic pain is a variant of anxiety. Certain conditions have been identified, however, such as tension headache, for which a significant aetiological contribution from anxiety has been generally accepted.

Fear avoidance leading to disability has begun to receive attention in the literature. Such constructions are consistent with the clinical observations of the present author, and are considered in greater detail in Chapter 9.

Merskey et al (1987), using the Irritability/Depression and Anxiety Questionnaire, found that 37% of 387 chronic pain patients were pathologically anxious. Perhaps anxiety is frequently

unrecognized in chronic pain, because the symptoms are attributed to the pain condition or to minor depression. Atkinson et al (1986) found no cases of anxiety disorders in 52 chronic pain patients. In an extensive review of chronic back pain Fishbain (1999) found a prevalence of anxiety disorders higher than expected for the general population.

Personality disorder

Merskey (1992) described the selection process preceding presentation at the pain clinic. Faced with chronic non-terminal pain, many individuals will tolerate the condition and get on with their normal activities as best as they can. Some will take over-the-counter medicines. Only a proportion will consult their general practitioner, and a small number of these will keep returning to the doctor after initial examination, reassurance and conservative treatment. Those who reach the pain clinic are a tiny, highly filtered and selected population. For those patients who reach the chronic pain clinic with similar physical pathology to those who do not, other factors, including personality features, may drive the presentation.

Friedman et al (1963) described a 'demanding, hypochondrical' form of depression. In most instances, this reflects depression in an individual with demanding and hypochondrical personality features.

Pilowsky et al (1977) compared pain clinic

patients to family medicine clinic patients using the Illness Behavior Questionnaire and found that pain patients demonstrated significantly more 'disease conviction' and 'somatic preoccupation' and were significantly more likely to 'deny life problems unrelated to their physical problem'. These features set the scene for a patient–doctor relationship that is unsatisfactory to both participants.

Somatizing and chronic pain patients are described as critical and unrewarding patients to manage, and unpopular with many clinicians (Barsky et al, 1991). They have been characterized as querulous, self-preoccupied, demanding and irritable (Engel, 1959).

Fishbain et al (1986) examined 283 patients using the DSM-III and found 62.3% of men and 55.1% of women merited a diagnosis of personality disorder. In a recent review of the field, Weisberg (2000) found that personality disorders are significantly greater in the pain population than in the general population or in medical or psychiatric populations.

Conclusion

Chronic pain is rarely cured. The reasonable aim is to relieve symptoms as much as possible. It is not clear that chronic pain is frequently accompanied by psychiatric disorder. Given our limited ability to assist those with chronic pain we should take every opportunity to relieve distress, this includes looking for and treating concurrent psychiatric disorders whenever they are detected.

References

Atkinson J, Ingram R, Kremer E, Saccuzzo D. MMPI subgroups and affective disorder in chronic pain patients. *Journal of Nervous and Mental Disease* 1986; 174: 408–13.

Barsky A, Wyshak G, Latham K, Klerman G. Hypochondrical patients, their physicians, and their medical care. *Journal of Internal Medicine* 1991; 6: 413–19.

Blumer D, Heilbronn M. Chronic pain as a variant of depressive disease. The pain-prone disorder. *Journal of Nervous and Mental Disorders* 1982; 170: 381–406.

Davidson J, Krishhnan R, France R, Pelton S. Neurovegetative symptoms in chronic pain and depression. *Journal of Affective Disorders* 1985; 9: 213–18.

Dworkin R, Gitlin M. Clinical aspects of depression in chronic pain patients. *Clinical Journal of Pain* 1991; 7: 79–94.

Engel G. 'Psychogenic' pain and the pain-prone patient. *American Journal of Medicine* 1959; 26: 899–918.

Fishbain D. Approaches to treatment decisions for psychiatric comorbidity in management of the chronic pain patient. *Medical Clinics of North America* 1999; 83: 737–60.

Fishbain D, Goldberg M, Meager B, Rosomoff H. Male and female chronic pain patients categorized by DSM-III criteria. *Pain* 1986; 26: 181–97.

Fishbain D, Cutler R, Rosomoff H. Chronic pain associated depression: antecedent or consequence of chronic pain? A review. *Clinical Journal of Pain* 1997; 13: 79–87.

Friedman A, Cowitz B, Cowen H, Gramick S. Syndromes and themes of psychiatric depression. *Archives of General Psychiatry* 1963; 9: 504–9.

Merskey H. Chronic pain problems and psychiatry. In: Tyrer S (ed) *Psychology, Psychiatry and Chronic Pain*. Butterworth Heinemann, Oxford, 1992; 45–56.

Merskey H, Lau C, Russell E, Brooke R, James M, Lappano S, Neilsoen J, Tilsworth R. Screening for psychiatric morbidity. The pattern of psychological illness and premorbid characteristics in four chronic pain populations. *Pain* 1987; 30: 141–57.

Pilowsky I, Chapman C, Bonica J. Pain depression and illness behavior in a pain clinic population. *Pain* 1977; 4: 183–92.

Roth R. Psychogenic models of chronic pain: a selective review and critique. In: Massie MJ (ed) *Pain: What Psychiatrists Need to Know*. (Review of Psychiatry Series, Vol. 19, No 2, Oldham J and Riba M, series eds). American Psychiatric Press, Washington, DC, 2000; 89–131.

Sullivan M, Reesor K, Mikail S, Fisher R. The treatment of depression in chronic low back pain: review and recommendations. *Pain* 1992; 50: 5–13.

Turk D, Flor H. Etiological theories and treatments for chronic back pain. II Psychological models and interventions. *Pain* 1984; 19: 209–33.

Weisberg J. Personality and personality disorders in chronic pain. *Current Review of Pain* 2000; 4: 60–70.

Wise M, Taylor S. Anxiety and mood disorders in medically ill patients. *Journal of Clinical Psychiatry* 1990; 51: 27–32.

Pain and somatization

*'Our doctor would never really operate unless it was necessary.
If he didn't need the money, he wouldn't lay a hand on you'*
Herb Shriner

One of the great challenges faced by medical practitioners is the care of people who complain of physical symptoms for which no physical cause, or only insufficient physical cause, can be found. This problem has a long history. When observed in the women of ancient Greece it was believed that the womb (*hystera*) of the patient was roaming within her body, and the condition was called 'hysteria'. When a person believed that he or she had an illness for which there was no evidence the term 'hypochondria' was employed, which indicated that the problem was under the cartilage (chondrium) of the front of the chest.

Overlapping conditions

Somatization

Somatization is defined (Lipowski, 1988) as the propensity to experience and report somatic symptoms that have no pathophysiological explanation, to misattribute them to disease, and to seek medical attention for them. The elements of this definition deserve individual examination. There is a 'propensity': thus particular personality traits or beliefs are present and repetition of the behaviour can be expected. The symptoms are 'experienced', not just reported. Thus, somatizing patients are not feigning symptoms, and somatization is distinct from factitious disorder and malingering. There is no 'pathophysiological explanation' to be found in the organ or region in which such a finding could be expected; however, comorbid psychiatric symptoms may exist. The misattribution of symptoms to disease may result in, or in cases of longer standing, arise out of, the belief that disease is present. There is ample opportunity for misattribution, as population-based surveys reveal that healthy adults experience more than one somatic symptom each week (Egan and Beaton, 1987). Medical attention is sought and sought frequently; however, this may be insignificant in comparison to the attention sought from relatives, friends, pharmacist and alternative therapists.

This is a descriptive account, free of aetiological speculation. Others (Shapiro, 1965; Schalling et al, 1973), using neuropsychological testing, have shown that somatization is associated with information-processing deficits. A current review has confirmed that such patients manifest specific cognitive features (Rief and Nanke, 1999).

Alexithymia, which means being 'without words to describe emotions', has also been reported to be an important factor (Sifneos, 1996). It is proposed that, in the absence of the ability to describe emotions, individuals respond to life situations in maladaptive ways. Alexithymic individuals focus on facts, details and external events, and tend to have a limited fantasy life.

Many individuals who do not satisfy strict diagnostic criteria for alexithymia nevertheless have an impoverished ability to express their emotions in words or by other adaptive means. Important factors include intelligence, education and culture/sub-culture (e.g. 'macho' males). Somatization is more frequent in the lower socioeconomic classes, where opportunities are limited (Gentry et al, 1974). Also important, once the patient has presented, is the ability of the patient and the doctor to communicate effectively. Here, much responsibility rests with the doctor, who must attend and work to understand the patient's 'physical' language.

Somatization disorder

Somatization disorder as defined in DSM-IV (APA, 1994) remains a controversial diagnosis. Somatization (the process) as described by Lipowski does occur in somatization disorder; but the presence of the process is not sufficient to justify the diagnosis. For somatization disorder there must be a lifetime history of pain in at least four different parts of the body and at least one conversion or dissociative symptom.

In hysteria, an earlier designation for this disorder, using neuropsychological testing, information-processing deficits were demonstrated. These were characterized by distractibility and difficulty in distinguishing target stimuli (Ludwig, 1972; Flor-Henry et al, 1981).

Hypochondriasis

Hypochondriasis (DSM-IV) involves preoccupation with an unrealistic fear or belief of having a serious disease, despite negative investigation and assurance that no relevant pathophysiology is present. Fear or belief of having a serious disease, however, is common to all somatoform disorders. There are doubts as to whether hypochondriasis is a discrete disease entity (Rief et al, 1998). The diagnosis is frequently made in the primary care setting. Management is notoriously difficult.

The DSM-IV can be criticized for giving a new definition to an old problem. Many older textbooks (Curran and Partridge, 1969) did not list hypochondriasis as a discrete entity, instead, indexing it 'in endogenous depression, in GPI, in involutional melancholia, in schizophrenia, in senescence'. Kenyon (1976) has strongly argued that hypochondriasis is always a secondary part of another syndrome, usually a depressive disorder.

In the earlier diagnostic systems that did allow hypochondriasis as a discrete entity, hypochondrical thoughts could be held with delusional intensity. Using the DSM-IV system, when delusions are present it is necessary to make the diagnosis of delusional disorder.

Pain disorder

Pain disorder associated with psychological factors or with both psychological factors and a general medical condition is distinct from somatization disorder in the DSM-IV system. However, some (Katon et al, 1984; Aigner and Bach, 1999) regard chronic pain as the most common form of somatization. The diagnosis of pain disorder is particularly difficult when there has been physical disease or injury due to incompletely understood phenomena, including sympathetically maintained pain (Walker and Cousins, 1997) and the painful joint stiffness and muscular weakness associated with disuse.

There is evidence that prior experience of pain can influence the response to stimuli (Bayer et al, 1998). Learning appears to be aetiologically important in pain disorder, as secondary gains reinforce pain-related behaviour; and prior social models, especially sick and suffering parents, predispose to the development of the condition (Apley, 1975). The factors that sustain chronic pain (particularly low back pain) probably include fear of movement and pain, which can lead to the disuse syndrome and a self-perpetuating cycle (Vlaeyen and Linton, 2000).

Conceptual underpinning

Attribution theory

What individuals believe about their symptoms greatly influences whom they consult and how they manage those symptoms (King, 1983). Individuals have enduring attributional styles (Garcia-Campayo et al, 1997), such that when a symptom is experienced, it is likely to be attributed to a physical, psychological or environmental/normalizing explanation (Robins and Kirmayer, 1991). Not surprisingly, general practice attenders with hypochondrical tendencies have more physical attributions than those with anxiety disorders (MacLeod et al, 1998). Educational programmes designed to modify attribution style are useful in the management of chronic pain and somatization.

Medical anthropology

Illness may be defined, anthropologically, as 'the human experience of sickness'. The process begins with personal awareness of a change in body feeling and continues with the labelling of the sufferer by self and family as 'ill' (Kleinman et al, 1978). Illness is greatly dependent on family and cultural beliefs about disease and discomfort, and is consequently culturally constructed (Wexler, 1974). It may be construed as the patient's view of clinical reality (patient's view). Some (Stimson, 1974) claim that medical doctors treat illness poorly, while traditional and alternative therapists, who listen and give culturally relevant explanations, treat illness well.

Disease may be defined as 'abnormalities in the structure and function of body organs and systems'. It may be construed at the medical view of clinical reality (medical view). One criticism of modern medicine is that it focuses on the treatment of disease and ignores the treatment of illness (Engel, 1977).

Common sense suggests a better outcome will be achieved if both illness and disease are treated. Toward this end, the doctor should seek to understand the patient's view fully, to explain the medical view and to negotiate a shared view (Von Korff et al, 1997).

Abnormal illness behaviour

Abnormal illness behaviour (AIB) provides an intellectual framework for a comprehensive range of human behaviours (Pilowsky, 1969). It depends on two sociological concepts: illness behaviour and the sick role. Illness behaviour is defined as 'the ways in which individuals experience, perceive, evaluate and respond to their own health status' (Mechanic, 1968). The sick role is conceptualized as bringing obligations and privileges (Parsons, 1964). The obligations are that the person seeking the role: (1) accepts that the role is undesirable; (2) co-operates with others to achieve health; and (3) utilizes the services of those regarded by society as competent in healing. If these obligations are fulfilled, the individual is granted the following privileges: (1) to be regarded as not being responsible for his/her condition; (2) to be accepted as someone requiring care; and (3) exempted from normal obligations (such as work).

On these foundations, Pilowsky (1997) defined AIB as 'an inappropriate or maladaptive mode of experiencing, evaluating or acting in relation to one's own state of health, which persists, despite the fact that a doctor (or other recognized social agent) offered accurate and reasonably lucid information concerning the person's health status and the appropriate course of management (if any), with provision of adequate opportunity for discussion, clarification and negotiation, based on a thorough examination of all parameters of functioning (physical, psychological and social) taking into account the individual's age, educational and sociocultural background'.

AIB is a multifaceted thesis of great theoretical importance. It highlights the connection between social influences and health and provides a unifying conceptual basis for illness-related behaviour, including but extending beyond the somatoform disorders to factitious disorder and malingering, and, in another direction, to the denial of illness. It casts the individual who denies illness and stays at work under the same umbrella as the individual who pretends illness and goes to the football – with the vast majority of illness behaviours lying somewhere between these two extremes.

In addition, AIB supplies the context for the responsibility of the doctor as the socially designated controller of sick role privileges, a frequently onerous and unwelcome duty.

Medicalization

Medicalization describes the tendency of contemporary society to focus attention on the medical aspects of everyday life. It shares roots with the principle of social justice, in an increasingly humane society. In general it places increased responsibilities with health professionals, health authorities and health insurers. This process is a feature of society, not of the individual. However, the constructs of society influence the course of action and options that will be chosen by the individual.

An example of one form of medicalization is the presentation at the general hospital of people with social problems. Marital disputes frequently result in one party's achieving admission to hospital, wrongly diagnosed as suffering a psychiatric disorder. Another form is an accompaniment of very sensible, well-intentioned public health endeavours such as those that urge people to take chest pain seriously and to be alert for the early signs of diabetes/cancer. In all probability these save lives. Just as probably, they encourage the public to regard every ache and pain as a warning sign of disease and an indication for medical examination.

The biopsychosocial model

The biopsychosocial model aims to take account of the broad range of influences (biological, psychological and social – cultural can also be included) that may coalesce in the formation of a disorder.

An example is provided by the consideration of chronic pain resulting from whiplash injury following rear-end collisions (Ferrari and Russell, 1999). The late whiplash syndrome is culturally constructed, being non-existent or almost non-existent in Singapore, Lithuania, Germany and Greece, and among laboratory volunteers and fairground bumper car revellers, but common in the USA and Australia. Evidence suggests that in England, whiplash replaced 'railway spine' (Trimble, 1981). The claimants are neither malingering nor suffering a psychiatric disorder.

In this example, the biological dimension is most probably an acute sprain, which resolves/heals without any significant residual structural damage. At least, no convincing,

enduring pathology has been demonstrated using current medical technology. Important psychosocial determinants are observed in cultures that provide 'overwhelming information' regarding the potential for chronic pain following whiplash injury, medical systems that encourage inactivity and caution, and litigation processes that involve protracted battles with insurance companies. Patients are led to expect, amplify and attribute symptoms in a chronic fashion.

Synthesis/summary

Lipowski's view that some individuals have a propensity to experience and report somatic symptoms that have no pathophysiological explanation, to misattribute them to disease, and to seek medical attention has not been disputed in the literature and can be accepted. Somatoform disorder, hypochondriasis and pain disorder remain contentious, in so far as they may not represent discrete disease entities. However, they all have elements of somatization and currently emerge in a setting of medicalization. Evidence suggests that cognitive processes may be aetiologically important. Both somatization and somatoform disorder are reported to be associated with information-processing deficits. In pain disorder learning appears to be an aetiological factor; there is evidence supporting the influence of secondary gains and social models. Fear of pain and movement may be important in the maintenance of some chronic pain.

Other support for the importance of cognition in somatization and somatization disorder is available. Attributional theory is not yet firmly established, but advances the reasonable proposition that ambiguous symptoms will be interpreted in accordance with personal beliefs and experience. Medical anthropology emphasizes the importance of the beliefs of the individual and the culture. The sociological concepts mentioned here impact on classification rather than aetiology. AIB forms an alternative envelope for certain DSM-IV disorders, and does not obstruct the proposal that cognitive factors are of aetiological importance. Whiplash disorder is an example of a chronic, painful, incapacitating syndrome that is secondary to the cognitions of the patient, plus those of the society and culture in general, and the medical and legal professions in particular. (With respect to chronic pain, fear of movement and pain may serve to perpetuate this condition via the disuse syndrome.)

Management recommendations

1. The anthropologists inform us that there are at least two views of clinical reality (the patient's and the medical view) and that the best outcome is achieved when the patient and doctor can discuss their respective belief systems and come to a shared view of clinical reality. Others have made similar observations. This approach is recommended.

2. The evidence for information-processing deficits in these clinical presentations suggests that information should be presented in an understandable form and repeated frequently. The presence of information-processing deficits is one reason why such patients may not respond to the advice and information in the same manner as might other patients. This knowledge may reduce the burden of their care.

3. Present at all times as caring, confident, firm and approachable (within agreed limits).

4. After appropriate investigation, inform the patient that no further investigations are indicated, at this time. Investigations are expensive, dangerous and usually unhelpful. Reassure that investigations will be conducted, in the future, as indicated.

5. Limit the number of invasive treatments.

6. Limit the number of doctors the patient consults. The limitation of investigations and invasive treatments is only possible when there is a limit on the number of doctors involved in the case. Continue to be involved on condition that the patient does not go outside the agreed team. An interested general practitioner is

essential. In the case of somatization, somatization disorder and hypochondriasis, a combination of an interested general practitioner and a consulting psychiatrist, who are able to communicate as necessary, is recommended. In the case of pain disorder, a combination of an interested general practitioner and a consulting psychiatrist or pain medicine specialist, who are able to communicate as necessary, is recommended.

7. Limit the time spent with the patient. Do not present this as a punitive issue. Rather, discuss the fact that the patient's needs can best be met by regularly scheduled time-defined appointments. Point out that you are prepared to help, but that this is only possible if meetings are regularized. Negotiate a sensible protocol to be followed in the case of crises.

8. The patient has the right to care. Attention may be according to a time schedule, but should not be contingent on the patient's suppressing or hiding pain behaviour.

9. Limit the amount of medication. Benzodiazepines, stimulants and analgesics should be strenuously limited. These patients do experience distress, and the use of antidepressants and mood stabilizers has a role. Antipsychotic medication has a place in highly aroused individuals or where psychosis is observed or suspected.

10. Analgesics should be taken on a regular basis. The taking of medication 'as required' reinforces pain behaviour by providing sudden rewarding pain relief, and in the worst case scenario, a 'rush', in response to the taking of a pill. This is not to prohibit the patient on long-acting medication from taking small additional amounts for 'breakthrough' pain.

11. Diagnose and adequately treat comorbid psychiatric disorders.

12. Provide some emotional support. Chronic pain patients suffer emotionally as well as physically.

13. Encourage return to normal activities. This is the best way to combat pain-related fear that leads to the disuse syndrome and cyclical pain. Encourage hobbies, exercise, education and cultural pursuits – these will distract the patient from his/her body, stretch and strengthen the body and assist the return to normal function. Reward attempts at activities with praise.

(The joints and muscles stiffen during prolonged inactivity. The return to activity must be graded and gradual, but relentless. The active patient should take frequent rests. Activity that is overzealous may result in the exacerbation of symptoms. This in turn may lead to further patient-imposed bed rest and the avoidance of activity. In chronic painful conditions, pain usually does not indicate further damage.)

14. Educate and involve the family in management.

15. Understand the need to repeat the reassurance, encouragement of activities and conditions of care (the limits).

References

Aigner M, Bach M. Clinical utility of DSM-IV pain disorder. *Comprehensive Psychiatry* 1999; 40: 353–7.

APA (American Psychiatric Association). *Diagnostic and Statistical Manual of Mental Disorders*, 4th edn. American Psychiatric Association, Washington, DC, 1994.

Apley J. *The Child With Abnormal Pains*. Blackwell, Oxford, 1975.

Bayer T, Coverdale J, Chiang E, Bangs M. The role of prior pain experience and expectancy in psychologically and physically induced pain. *Pain* 1998; 74: 327–31.

Curran D, Partridge M. *Psychological Medicine*, 6th edn. E & S Livingstone, Edinburgh, 1969.

Egan K, Beaton R. Response to symptoms in health low utilisers of the health care system. *Journal of Psychosomatic Research* 1987, 31, 11–21.

Engel G. The need for a new medical model: a challenge for biomedicine. *Science* 1977; 196: 129–36.

Ferrari R and Russell A. Epidemiology of whiplash: an international dilemma. *Annals of the Rheumatic Diseases* 1999; 58: 1–5.

Flor-Henry P, Fromm-Auch D, Tapper M,

Schopflocher D. A neuropsychological study of the stable syndrome of hysteria. *Biological Psychiatry* 1981; 16: 601–627.

Garcia-Campayo J, Larrubia J, Lobo A, Perez-Echeverria M, Campos R. Attribution in somatizers: stability and relationship to outcome at 1-year follow-up. *Acta Psychiatrica Scandinavica* 1997; 95: 433–8.

Gentry W, Shows W, Thomas M. Chronic low back pain: a psychological profile. *Psychosomatics* 1974; 15: 174–7.

Katon W, Ries R, Kleinman A. The prevalence of somatization in primary care. *Comprehensive Psychiatry* 1984; 25: 208–15.

Kenyon F. Hypochondrical states. *British Journal of Psychiatry* 1976; 129: 1–14.

King F. Attribution theory and the health belief model. In: Hewstone M (ed) *Attribution Theory: Social and Functional Extensions*. Basil Blackwell, Oxford, 1983; 170–86.

Kleinman A, Eisenberg L, Good B. Clinical lessons from anthropologic and cross-cultural research. *Annals of Internal Medicine* 1978; 88: 251–8.

Lipowski Z. Somatization: the concept and its clinical applications. *American Journal of Psychiatry* 1988; 145: 1358–68.

Ludwig A. Hysteria: a neurobiological theory. *Archives of General Psychiatry* 1972; 27: 771–86.

MacLeod A, Haynes C, Sensky T. Attributions about common body sensations: their associations with hypochondriasis and anxiety. *Psychological Medicine* 1998; 28: 225–8.

Mechanic D. *Medical Sociology*. Free Press, New York, 1968.

Parsons T. *Social Structure and Personality*. Collier-Macmillan, London, 1964.

Pilowsky I. Abnormal illness behaviour. *British Journal of Medical Psychology* 1969; 42: 347–51.

Pilowsky I. *Abnormal Illness Behaviour*. John Wiley & Sons Ltd, Chichester, 1997.

Rief W, Nanke A. Somatization disorder from a cognitive-psychobiological perspective. *Current Opinion in Psychiatry* 1999; 12: 733–8.

Rief W, Hiller W, Margraf J. Cognitive aspects of hypochondriasis and the somatization syndrome. *Journal of Abnormal Psychology* 1998; 107: 587–95.

Robins J, Kirmayer L. Attributions of common somatic symptoms. *Psychological Medicine* 1991; 21: 1029–45.

Schalling D, Cronholm B, Asberg M, Espmark S. Rating of psychiatric and somatic anxiety incidents – interrater reliability and relations to personality variables. *Acta Psychiatrica Scandinavica* 1973; 49: 353–68.

Shapiro D. *Neurotic Styles*. Basic Books, New York, 1965.

Sifneos P. Alexithymia: past and present. *American Journal of Psychiatry* 1996; 153 (7 Suppl): 137–42.

Stimson G. Obeying the doctor's orders: a view from the other side. *Social Science Medicine* 1974, 8, 97–104.

Trimble M. *Post-traumatic Neurosis: From Railway Spine to the Whiplash*. Wiley, Chichester, 1981.

Vlaeyen J, Linton S. Fear-avoidance and its consequences in chronic musculoskeletal pain: a state of the art. *Pain* 2000; 85: 317–32.

Von Korff M, Gruman J, Schaefer J, Curray S, Wagner E. Collaborative management of chronic illness. *Annals of Internal Medicine* 1997; 127: 1097–102.

Walker S, Cousins M. Complex regional pain syndromes: including 'reflex sympathetic dystrophy' and 'causalgia'. *Anaesthesia and Intensive Care* 1997; 25: 113–25.

Wexler N. Culture and mental illness: a social labelling perspective. *Journal of Nervous and Mental Diseases* 1974; 159: 379–95.

Fear of movement and pain

9

> 'No passion so effectively robs the mind of all its powers of
> acting and reasoning as fear.'
>
> *Edmund Burke 1729–1797*

Fear of movement and pain (pain-related fear), leading to
avoidance, inactivity and disability, appears to be a factor in
the aetiology of some cases of chronic pain. The theory is
consistent with clinical experience and is supported by an
impressive body of research. The 'fear-avoidance model' of
chronic pain was first described by Lethem et al in 1983.
Recent reviews of the field are available (Asmundson et al,
1999; Crombez et al, 1999). The research has been mainly
concerned with low back pain; but in clinical practice pain-
related fear and consequent avoidance of activity is observed
with other chronic pain conditions.

Pain is the most aversive stimulus known to man.

It is reasonable to expect that patients who were
premorbidly anxious about health matters will be especially
susceptible to developing pain-related fear.

Fear of movement

Fear of activity may develop when pain has been experienced acutely, during activity. Warnings from doctors and other authorities to avoid activity or the witnessing of pain experienced by others while performing tasks may have similar effects. Both classical and operant learning may be involved (Vlaeyen and Linton, 2000). In so far as these patients cease normal functions, they are disabled.

Fear of pain

The fear of pain model is similar to the fear of movement model, but is more elaborate and is more concerned with cognitive processes (Waddell et al, 1993). In this model the patient has an inaccurate understanding of the pain and its consequences. When the patient believes that pain indicates damage, pain is feared and movements that cause pain are avoided. The patient needs to learn that, in acute pain situations, pain does indicate damage and activities that extend the pain may extend the damage. However, the chronic pain situation is different. Healing has taken place and the structure of the body is stable. In this situation pain does not indicate ongoing damage; in fact, the fear of pain and the avoidance of activity will delay the optimization of outcome.

The disuse syndrome

A consequence of the avoidance of movement is the disuse syndrome (Kottke, 1996). This includes the loss of muscle strength, increasing joint stiffness, lowering of the pain threshold and the impairment of muscle coordination. In clinical practice the impairment of muscle coordination takes the form of 'guarding' or prevention, by muscle contraction, of particular movements. The scene is thus set for a destructive cycle in which pain-related fear leads to further pain and so forth. Theoretically, at least, the process persists because extinction is delayed. As there is little movement there is little opportunity to learn that movement does not lead to unendurable pain.

Fear and cognitive functions

Fear increases vigilance. Once a patient has experienced pain-related fear, he/she is more likely to notice and place importance on minor pains and sensations and overestimate the importance of them.

Fear distracts and impairs concentration and thereby interferes with cognition. There is speculation that pain-related fear may interfere with the patient's ability fully to comprehend and accept information provided by health professionals, and to utilize information to change thinking and behaviour patterns. In particular, the effect of pain-related fear may be to impair the ability to accept that, in the chronic situation, pain does not mean further injury.

Clinical implications

Many aspects of pain-related fear have been confirmed, and formal screening of patients may become routine clinical practice.

At present, screening may be achieved using clinical skills. It is common for fearful patients to deny fear on initial, direct questioning. Matters become clearer if patients are asked to give an account of their understanding of the nature of their problem and the consequences of movement. It is important to know if patients anticipate immediate or delayed pain, or further injury.

A number of questionnaires may be useful in the identification process. Fear of pain has been measured using Pain And Impairment Relationship Scale (PAIRS: Riley et al, 1988) and the Pain Anxiety Symptoms Scale (PASS: McCracken et al, 1992). Fear of movement's causing further damage has been measured using the Survey Of Pain Attitudes (SOPA: Jensen et al, 1987) and the Tampa Scale for Kinesiophobia (TSK: Kori et al, 1990). Fear of work-related activities has been measured using the Fear Avoidance Beliefs Questionnaire (FABQ: Waddell et al, 1993). These may provide a screening role, but cut-off points indicating clinical significance have yet to be published.

Educational efforts can be focused on misunderstandings. Theoretically, correction of illogical thinking or catastrophizing could prevent or reduce pain-related fear, avoidance and disability.

The term 'cognitive behaviour therapy' has been applied to such patient–clinician interactions. This may discourage clinicians who lack such training. However, clear communication, accurate information and encouragement are central, and are skills possessed by all experienced clinicians.

Graded physical activity may be the most effective method of preventing and rehabilitating pain-related fear and disability (Vlaeyen et al, 2001). A recent advance in the management of acute back pain was the change from extended bed rest to early return to normal activities.

Graded physical activity makes particular sense where there is a phobia about pain and movement (McQuade et al, 1988). Also, there are people who are impervious to persuasion and who need to 'see things with their own eyes'. Finally, after a period of inactivity, those with chronic pain are likely to experience increased pain during the recommencement of activity. There may or may not be an eventual diminution of pain. What will be achieved in the vast majority of cases, however, is a decrease in disability. This is a frightening, worrying time, and the presence of an informed clinician who acknowledges that the task is difficult, but encourages perseverance, is a great advantage.

The best results can be expected when cognitive and physical approaches are combined in a supportive environment.

References

Asmundson G, Norton P, Norton G. Beyond pain: the role of fear and avoidance in chronicity. *Clinical Psychology Review* 1999; 19: 97–119.

Crombez G, Vlaeyen J, Heuts P, Lysens R. Pain-related fear is more disabling than pain itself. Evidence of the role of pain-related fear in chronic back pain disability. *Pain* 1999; 80: 329–40.

Jensen M, Karoly P, Huger R. The development and preliminary validation of an instrument to assess patients' attitudes toward pain. *Journal of Psychosomatic Research* 1987; 31: 393–400.

Kori S, Miller R, Todd D. Kinisophobia: a new view of chronic pain behavior. *Pain Management* 1990; Jan/Feb: 35–43.

Kottke F. The effects of limitation of activity upon the human body. *Journal of the American Medical Association* 1996; 196: 117–22.

Lethem J, Slade P, Troup J, Bentley G. Outline of fear-avoidance model of exaggerated pain perceptions. *Behavior Research Therapy* 1983; 21: 401–8.

McCracken L, Zayfert C, Gross R. The pain anxiety symptom scale: development and validation of a scale to measure the fear of pain. *Pain* 1992; 50: 63–7.

McQuade K, Turner J, Buchner D. Physical fitness and chronic low back pain. *Clinical Orthopaedics Related Research* 1988; 198–204.

Riley J, Ahern D, Follick M. Chronic pain and functional impairment: assessing beliefs about their relationship. *Archives of Physical Medicine and Rehabilitation* 1988; 69: 579–82.

Vlaeyen J, Linton S. Fear-avoidance and its consequences in chronic musculoskeletal pain: a state of the art. *Pain* 2000; 85: 317–32.

Vlaeyen J, de Jong J, Geilen M, Heuts P, van Breukelen G. Graded exposure in vivo in the treatment of pain-related fear: a replicated single-case experimental design in four patients with chronic low back pain. *Behavior Research Therapy* 2001; 39: 151–66.

Waddell G, Newton M, Henderson I, Somerville D, Main C. A Fear-Avoidance Beliefs Questionnaire (FABQ) and the role of fear-avoidance beliefs in chronic low back pain and disability. *Pain* 1993; 52: 157–68.

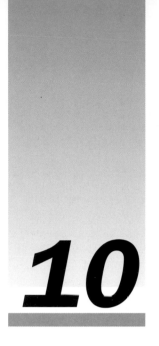

Relaxation, hypnosis and meditation

'The highest possible stage in moral culture is when we recognize that we ought to control our thoughts.'

Charles Darwin 1871

It is possible to gain some relief from the separate entities of anxiety and physical pain through the use of relaxation, hypnosis and meditation techniques. Physical pain is usually accompanied, and is always heightened, by anxiety or similar mental distress. Faced with the dilemma of chronic pain, these techniques should be exploited.

Overview of techniques

Relaxation is infrequently defined. It has been described as the absence of tension, stress, discomfort, anxiety and distress. It is a psychophysiological state (it has mental and physical components). The key features include increased slow brain wave activity, lowered respiration and heart rate, lowered adrenal outflow, and a lowering of mental activity other than effortless attention. A definition from scholars interested in response to stimuli reads 'A generalized psychophysiological, wakeful state of minimal activity or preparation for response to any demand placed upon the body and mind' (Wentworth-Rohr, 1988). Both components, mental and physical, must be targeted in the pursuit of the relaxed state.

Hypnosis also lacks a straightforward definition. It is swathed in mystique. It is known as a method by which deep trance states can be induced and potent post-hypnotic suggestions implanted. Importantly, to the present time, it lacks a physiological profile to distinguish it from relaxation. One definition of hypnosis is 'a consent state of physiological relaxation in which the critical faculty of the conscious mind is by-passed to some degree' (Scott, 1974). This purported distinguishing feature of hypnosis, the potential for by-passing 'the critical faculty of the conscious mind', may not be unique, however, as proponents of relaxation and meditation also claim to achieve increased receptivity to suggestion (Meares, 1968).

The difficulties of hypnosis include the stigma of charlatanism (the legacy of stage hypnotists) and the suspicion of malevolent mind control that pervade the public view. There is the difficulty of deciding whether or not a patient is a good hypnotic subject. There may be difficulty in inducing hypnosis; even patients who appear to be good candidates and have received adequate preparation may resist induction. Patients may claim that they were 'not really' hypnotized and were 'just pretending', a situation that calls for time-consuming exploration. There is

the risk of strong transference (Freud is said to have been unexpectedly kissed by a patient when she woke from a trance). There is also the risk of the hypnotist developing the 'Messiah Complex' (Scott, 1974).

These difficulties represent no challenge for the thoroughly trained hypnotherapist. For those without such training, however, they represent significant obstacles. The present account will borrow elements from hypnosis, but does not attempt a comprehensive coverage of that field.

Relaxation, hypnosis and meditation all have the potential to narrow concentration, focus attention and increase receptivity to suggestion. The common denominator is the reduction of physiological arousal and the removal of distressing thoughts.

Benefits persist

The relaxation, hypnosis and meditation treatments of anxiety and pain have not been extensively studied with the randomized, double blind, placebo-controlled trials that characterize medication treatment research. Nevertheless, various relaxation procedures have earned a place as effective treatments of these conditions.

When a patient is physically and mentally relaxed, there can be little anxiety and mental distress. Proponents of relaxation, hypnosis and meditation tell us that with daily practice the benefits experienced during active treatment sessions begin to persist after the sessions have ceased. Over time these benefits last for longer and longer periods, until they remain throughout the entire day.

General technical details

The therapist should learn by undergoing instruction or attending classes whenever available. However, it is possible to learn sufficiently from books and personal experimentation to be able to offer patients some simple techniques.

It is better to avoid the use of the term 'hypnosis', which generates fear in some patients and may cause others to twist therapy into a contest of wills. Do not hesitate to involve a chaperon or friend/relative of the patient. Exercises for the body are an accepted feature of modern society. Relaxation, hypnosis and meditation are exercises for the mind and should be conduced in a similar, open (but confidential) matter-of-fact manner.

In the skill-acquisition stage (the first month) a technique should be practised as often as possible. This may be five or six times per day. The actual number of times this happens depends on enthusiasm and opportunity. Each practice session can be short: perhaps three to five minutes. It is better to persist until a noticeable change occurs, such as a change in rate of pulse or breathing or a sense of emotional peace. This indicates that appropriate processes have been initiated. With each initiation, ability increases. In the maintenance stage (after the first month) the technique should be practised every day. Some would say twice a day, but that may be unrealistic. A minimum of 20 minutes per day (total) should be so dedicated. With practice, ability to initiate relaxation increases and the total time necessary for good effect may be reduced.

In general, it is better for the patient to sit on a dining-style chair without arms or head rest, with feet flat on the floor and hands resting on the thighs. The relaxation sought is not like that which precedes sleep, and patients do not fall off their chairs. There are advantages to providing less than full body support; when sitting as described, it is necessary to work hard at achieving relaxation. Some authorities recommend a head rest; and it is possible to achieve relaxation in the supine position.

The patient usually sits with eyes lightly closed. This is not essential, as it is possible to achieve relaxation with the eyes open. When deep relaxation is achieved, the eyes may partially open. In the early skill-acquisition stage the patient may be troubled by trembling eyelids, but this passes within a week or so.

The therapist should speak in a quiet flat voice, similar to that used to deliver a sermon. Speaking slowly gives the patient time to perform the indicated tasks and the therapist time to decide on the next instruction. The therapist should repeat instructions for the same reasons.

Permissive phraseology should be employed. Use of commands ('You must relax your legs') will discourage co-operation and will usually result in failure of therapy. Some confident hypnotherapists use predictions ('Your finger will lift') to good effect. These predictions may be relying on little-known normal human physiology – for example, relaxed fingers do twitch from time to time – or on the power of suggestion, which may be facilitated by charisma, training and a good sense of timing. The term 'maybe' lacks confidence and is unlikely to be successful. The word 'can' ('See if you can slow your breathing still further') places the task with the patient.

Certain words, such as 'calm', 'drift', 'peace', 'sink', 'ease' and 'heavy', are favoured, as they not only impart information, but also strike a psychological cord that helps in triggering the desired response. New therapists develop their own lexicons and scripts with which they have success.

Patients should be informed of the need for regular practice. Relaxation sessions will be followed by periods of tranquillity, and the length of these periods will increase with practice. Sleep should also improve after a few days. Benefit during the day may be apparent at one week and will increase indefinitely. Patients need to be warned of the risk of a dip in motivation following the early honeymoon phase. Brief periods of even a few seconds of heaviness of limbs or drifting free of everyday thoughts during relaxation sessions are evidence that a favourable result can be achieved. Patients should be informed that, from this point, abilities and rewards rapidly become apparent.

Whether relaxation, hypnosis or meditation is achieved depends on the quality of the instructions of the therapist and the abilities of the patient. It is a given that treatment sessions are only attempted in safe, warm, suitably lit environments. The information made available by the therapist is standard information. From the outset it must be made clear that whether the desired endpoint is reached depends not on the abilities of the therapist, but on the abilities of the patient to follow and apply that information. This relieves the therapist of responsibility, and leaves it with the patient.

In handing this responsibility to the patient, the therapist should remember that a minority of people lack the ability to perform these activities and that these people must be protected from a sense of failure. Thus from the outset it is necessary to affirm that some people are good at some things and other people are good at other things. Some people are good at arithmetic, some are good at dancing and others are good at relaxation in therapists' offices. No one is good at everything, and some people are not particularly good at this form of relaxation. These people may be able to find relief in activities such as swimming or playing computer games. The point can be made that a mantra is (usually) a meaningless utterance that is useful because it allows participants to focus attention, and that a squash ball moving around on white walls, or a prompt blinking on a computer game screen can, at least in part, perform the role of the mantra, allowing freedom from intrusive concerns.

Before concluding that the patient can gain nothing from office-based relaxation techniques, however, it is obligatory for the therapist to offer more than a single method. To this end, some alternatives are described below.

Methods of focusing attention

Central to these techniques is the exclusion from the mind of worry and distressing thoughts. This may be achieved by occupying the mind with a task. It is possible to displace distressing thoughts with happy thoughts; but in the initiation stage of relaxation, hypnosis and meditation, it is better to use a neutral task. By focusing attention (concentrating) on the neutral task, awareness not only of worries and distress, but of the environment in general, is reduced, and the mind becomes less critical and more open to imagery, suggestion and autosuggestion. When the mind wanders

off the task and unbidden thoughts enter, they are not pushed away, but they are not attended and are allowed to pass through and away. The patient maintains a passive mental attitude, the only mental activity being the effortless focusing and refocusing of attention on the neutral task.

The mantra is a traditional Eastern mechanism. It is usually a sound that is repeated aloud or experienced silently. It becomes the focus of attention. These devices are used as an aid in many popular forms of meditation. Mantras share some of the features of counting sheep when sleep is evasive.

Focusing attention on breathing is a neutral task that is used in most if not all forms of relaxation, hypnosis and meditation. Most commonly the patient is asked to slow the breathing and to breathe with the diaphragm rather than the ribs. (In diaphragmatic breathing, as the diaphragm descends, and air enters the lungs, the anterior abdominal wall, rather than the chest wall, moves outward.) The patient may also be asked to focus on the flow and feel of the air as it enters the nose, trachea and lungs. In some relaxation and hypnosis techniques attention to breathing is alternated with attention to muscle relaxation. In some meditation techniques attention to breathing (the counting to 10 breaths and then starting again) is the only task (Wilson, 1995).

Focusing attention on the muscles is a

neutral task that was pioneered by Jacobson (1938). Like focusing on breathing, focusing on muscle relaxation achieves two ends simultaneously: it achieves one of the components of relaxation (decreased muscle tension) and it provides a focus for attention, thereby assisting the avoidance of worry and the thoughts of everyday living.

Special technical details

'Visualization' here means the formation of a mental image as though objects were being seen through the eyes. This process can be used either to initiate or to deepen the relaxed state or for both. The patient is asked to 'see' an image, often a serene water view. The patient must strongly focus to perform this task. The task can be made more exacting by asking the patient to 'see' things in greater detail. The therapist may ask: 'Try to see some small stones over to one side.' As a means of encouraging continued participation the therapist may ask the patient to indicate by lifting an index finger when some particular object can be 'seen' (details given below). Other perceptual modalities can be included. The patient may be asked to try to 'hear' waves or lapping water. The patient may be asked to 'smell' flowers. A particularly useful task is to ask the patient to 'feel' the warmth of the sun on the face. Patients may also be asked to 'see' themselves in and 'feel' the rocking of a rowing boat while visualizing a beach scene.

Another perceptual exercise that is mainly used to deepen relaxation is creating the experience of going down steps. Once some degree of relaxation is achieved the patient can be asked to see three steps leading down from their present position. The patient can be asked to indicate when this task has been achieved. Patients are then asked to 'feel' themselves move down from the top to the second step. As this occurs the patients are asked to feel themselves 'go deeper into relaxation'. The patient may be asked to indicate when this task has been achieved, and then to take the next step and go even deeper into the relaxed state. The number of steps can be altered to suit the therapist and the patient.

Ego-strengthening exercises have been described in the hypnosis literature. Once hypnosis is induced the hypnotherapist makes encouraging statements to the effect that the patient will become more confident, capable and contented. It is unlikely that this procedure modifies the ego as originally intended. However, having relaxed patients relive events in which they were appreciated and achieved positive results can serve as a task on which to focus, and simultaneously as a means of providing comfort and support. It is necessary to discover in preliminary discussion whether such an event can be identified. It is unhelpful to place this task before deeply relaxed patients if they are unable to identify events about which they have positive memories and feelings. The Stein (1963) clenched fist technique may be useful. Relaxed patients are asked to re-experience an event associated with positive thoughts and feelings; they are then asked to make a fist and 'keep hold' of those feelings. The hand is kept closed until after completion of the relaxation or hypnosis session. With practice, it is claimed that closing the hand outside relaxation sessions may trigger the desired experience.

It is possible to communicate with deeply relaxed patients by asking them to indicate answers by the voluntary raising of the index finger of one hand. This does not cause disturbance of the relaxed state. (Experts in hypnosis have described using the raising of a finger as a means of communicating with the unconscious; but that is a different matter.) Questions can be phrased such that they require yes or no answers, one hand answering, yes, and the other, no. This feature should not be overused, as it can have some temporary effect on the depth of relaxation. It can be used to good effect as a means of indicating when a task has been achieved, as in 'When you have been able to experience the feeling of inner peace, lift your index finger of your right hand.' Such phraseology increases the chance of success when the therapist is confident and positive: it is not a question of whether, but when the task will be achieved.

A valuable tool is to ask patients not only to follow instructions on an intellectual level,

but also to experience the associated feelings and emotions. For example, as mentioned above, the patient who is asked to slow the rate of breathing may also be asked to note the feeling of air going through the respiratory passages. A more complex task is for the patient who is asked to assume a peaceful attitude not simply to think of the concept of peace, but also to achieve the feeling or emotion of peace. These are more difficult tasks that require a greater degree of concentration and provide a deeper level of relaxation.

Semantic and mystical issues arise. There is no emotion called 'peace'. It is possible to feel peaceful; but patients may be asked to go beyond 'peaceful'. They may be asked to 'become' peace (for example), to allow their body and mind, identity or essence to be transformed into or blend with nature, God, the cosmos, or a universal serenity. At a more secular level, patients may usefully be asked to acquire or 'get' the feeling of drifting. It is better for therapists to remain on the secular side of the border with mysticism. From the medical perspective and in medical parlance such tasks foster a dissociative state. Dissociation is poorly defined, but includes the separation of ordinarily integrated behaviour, thought, feeling and consciousness. Thus, in so far as relaxation aims at producing a state of profound physical inactivity, avoidance of the present environment, and uncritical thought processes, there are similarities to a dissociative state. Relaxation of the type described here could be considered as controlled dissociation.

Complications of relaxation are very few. There is some danger of uncontrolled dissociation following treatment sessions. These are averted by discussion following treatments. The therapist ensures that the patient is orientated in time and place and restored to normal consciousness. Positive or negative experiences need to be reviewed, and the patient should be able to respond to potentially dangerous painful conditions in the appropriate manner.

Audiotapes may be made of relaxation sessions for use by patients at other times. This gives the patients an accurate account of the session and the opportunity to practise the tasks at their own pace. A potential disadvantage is that patients may become dependent on the therapist rather than developing their own initiative and self-administered relaxation sessions. Opinions differ from one therapist to another and one from one patient to another.

Developing a unique method

It is recommended that therapists should borrow from different techniques and develop a unique relaxation method with which they are personally comfortable and that suits their clinical circumstances.

Borrowing and modifying is well established in this field. For example, the original progressive muscular relaxation technique (Jacobson, 1938) called for repeated muscular contraction and relaxation of individual muscles or muscle groups, with whole sessions being spent on small anatomical areas and coverage of the whole body taking many weeks. Abbreviated versions were appropriated. More recent relaxation techniques have dispensed with the forceful contraction of muscles; instead, the attention of patients is directed to individual muscle groups, with the instruction simply to relax them during slow expiration. Different authors have drawn attention to the importance of relaxing different muscle groups (face, neck, hands); this appears to be a matter of personal preference.

Suggestion (defined for present purposes) is a primitive process by which ideas can be accepted into the mind without critical evaluation. Autosuggestion occurs when the subjects present ideas to themselves. These procedures were first described in hypnosis. However, as relaxation techniques also focus attention and increase receptivity, self-delivered ego-strengthening exercises, and positive self-messages, which constitute autosuggestion by other names, have been included in many relaxation protocols.

The relaxation technique described by Meares (1968) borrows from meditation techniques. The patient repeats thoughts: 'It is good to relax. Relaxing is natural. It is the natural way to calm and ease.' This is reminiscent of the repetition of a mantra. There is a difference, however, as these thoughts contain messages describing the desired mental state, which is not the case with most mantras.

Relaxation treatment of anxiety

Anxiety is common in pain states, and anxiety increases the suffering associated with pain. For these reasons it is appropriate to reduce anxiety in pain states. Relaxation (Fisher and Durham, 1999), hypnosis (Ashton et al, 1997) and meditation (Miller et al, 1995) have all been shown to reduce anxiety. The system described in this essay is a hybrid, elements having been drawn from across this therapeutic spectrum.

Relaxation, hypnosis and meditation are frequently practised by healthy individuals whose motives are many, including pleasure, self-development and self-awareness. No specific anti-anxiety component needs to be added for these to be considered effective treatments of anxiety. Obviously, these techniques produce a physical and mental state that is the antithesis of anxiety, and this is presumably relevant to their therapeutic action.

Patients can be taught to relax using scripts similar to the one that follows. They are encouraged to self-direct themselves through a similar process (this would be called autohypnosis, if the therapy were considered to be hypnosis) for a total of not less than 20 minutes per day. Patients are advised that there may be minor setbacks, but progress can be anticipated. Patients are also advised of the risk of loss of enthusiasm, particularly if progress is slower than desired.

The following scripts are provided as a guide to the types of relaxation sessions that can be developed. The therapist is encouraged to explore and modify.

Script 1
The following monologue gives an idea of a relaxation session early in the treatment/education process. Some repetition is given here, but in reality in a session lasting more than 10 minutes even more repetition would occur. In the initial phase of this session the focus is mainly on the musculature. That is not mandatory. Then the imagery of going down steps is used to deepen the relaxation. The patient is asked to communicate with the therapist using finger movements. Toward the end, encouraging statements are made and the patient is encouraged to remain in touch with positive feelings on cessation of the session.

> Please close your eyes . . . and try to follow my suggestions . . . I can tell you the things to aim for . . . but you are the one who has to do the work . . . First try to

concentrate on slowing your breathing down . . . Calm, slow breathing . . . Calm and relaxed . . . That's good . . . Now I want you to think about the muscles of your forehead . . . Let the muscles of your forehead relax . . . Calm, slow breathing . . . Calm and relaxed . . . As you breathe out say 'Relax', inside . . . Thinking of the muscles of your forehead . . . as you breathe out think, 'Relax' . . . Let the muscles of your forehead relax . . . Now think of the muscles of your face . . . your eyes . . . and your mouth . . . as you breath out say, 'Relax' . . . and let the muscles of your eyes . . . your face . . . and your mouth, relax . . . You are doing very well . . . You have control of your breathing . . . Now think of the muscles of your neck and shoulders . . . Relax your neck and shoulders . . . feel them sag a little . . . feel them sink . . . feel them heavy and relaxed . . . Calm and relaxed . . . Think of the muscles of your chest and your abdomen . . . let them relax . . . deeply relax . . . Now think of the muscles of your legs . . . as you breathe out . . . let your legs relax . . . Now think of your feet . . . Now think of your hands . . . as you breathe out . . . let your feet and hands relax . . . Calm and relaxed . . . Everything is heavy and relaxed . . . You are feeling good . . . You sink into the chair . . . You have done very well . . . I am going to stop talking for a minute . . . In the silence,

retain and explore this relaxed feeling for yourself.

OK, that's fine . . . You have calmed your breathing and relaxed . . . Well done . . . Now try to see three steps in front of you . . . Calm and relaxed . . . See yourself standing on the top step . . . with a path at the bottom . . . See the details of these three steps . . . Slow your breathing down . . . Very slow now . . . When you can see three steps . . . slowly move the index finger of your right hand.

OK, that's great . . . Now see if you can get the feeling of stepping down from the top step to the second step . . . Feeling good . . . Calm and relaxed . . . as you step down try to get the feeling of going deeper into relaxation . . . Try to get that feeling of stepping down . . . I will let you concentrate on stepping down . . . Move that finger when you have been able to get down.

Good . . . Now can you get down to the next step? . . . As you go down you will become more relaxed . . . Calm and relaxed . . . You are doing very well . . . Move your index finger when you have stepped down.

That's good . . . OK . . . Why don't you try to step down on to the path? . . . You have done very well . . . We will only go as far at the path today . . . Try to step down on to the path . . . As you do . . . feel yourself go even deeper into relaxation . . .

Heavy and sinking into the chair . . . Face relaxed . . . Neck relaxed . . . Chest relaxed . . . Legs relaxed . . . See if you can step down on to the path . . . As you step down you will get more relaxed than ever . . . Move that finger when you make it down to the path.

Well done. You should feel very pleased with yourself . . . You have taken control of your mind and your body . . . You are in control . . . Take a moment to explore the feeling of relaxation . . . take note that you have produced this state of profound relaxation . . . Let me know when you have been able to get a good feeling about what you have achieved.

OK, now we are going to start to come back up . . . Slowly turn around . . . See the steps in front of you . . . Keep hold of that good feeling about yourself . . . First, step back up one step . . . Feeling good . . . Calm and relaxed . . . Now back to the next step . . . Holding on to that good feeling . . . Now finally up to the top step . . . You have done very well . . . You have taken control of your mind and body . . . Gradually let your eyes open . . . Hold on to that good feeling . . . Don't move too fast . . . You have been deeply relaxed . . . You have been in control . . . You have done well.

OK. How do you feel?

Script 2

This monologue demonstrates the initiation

of relaxation by focusing on breathing. In a preliminary discussion it is necessary to establish whether the patient is able to breathe through the nose. If not, it is necessary to modify the wording to detail breathing through the mouth. In this discussion it will also be necessary to determine whether the patient is capable of diaphragmatic breathing. If not, a lesson will be necessary. Finally, it will be necessary to discover a happy event in the life of the patient. This is preferably an event in which the patient played an active part. The preferred event was marked by the patient's feeling capable and appreciated. It is used as a visualization task and a means of making supportive statements.

Please close your eyes and focus on your breathing . . . breathe in through your nose . . . Feel the air going into your nostrils . . . Slow the flow down . . . Concentrate only on your breathing . . . Concentrate on your nostrils . . . Feel the air cool and flowing freely . . . Now let yourself relax . . . Think of the air going down your neck . . . Flowing freely . . . Slow your breathing . . . Feel the air go into your chest . . . You can relax . . . Feel your body heavy and relaxed in the chair . . . As the air enters your body . . . Feel your tummy rise . . . Relax your chest . . . Let your chest be heavy . . . When the air comes into your body . . . let your tummy rise . . . Your breathing is much slower now . . . Your tummy rises very slowly . . . You can hardly feel it rise . . . Relaxed all over . . . I will stop talking for a minute and let you concentrate on your slow relaxed breathing.

Great, you're doing fine . . . You are in control . . . Check your body . . . If you have tension anywhere . . . Let go . . . See if you can get the feeling of drifting . . . As if you are floating . . . Drifting . . . Let go and drift.

Now get in touch with that time we were talking about . . . See yourself in that situation . . . See the details . . . Let yourself drift . . . Now get in touch with that feeling of success . . . Get that feeling of being pleased . . . Get that feeling of confidence . . . Things went well . . . Hold on to that feeling of success . . . Let yourself drift . . . I am going to be quiet now for a minute and let you get those feelings flowing over you.

Good. Now, hold on to that feeling as you come back . . . Gradually coming up . . . hold on to that feeling . . . Feeling calm . . . Feeling Good.

How do you feel now?

Relaxation treatment of pain

Relaxation (NIH, 1996), hypnosis (Lang et al, 2000) and meditation (Kaplan et al, 1993) have been shown to reduce pain. Reduction in chronic pain (Lewis, 1992) may be achieved using exactly the same techniques used in the treatment of anxiety. Hypnosis is used in acute dentistry, burns and surgery. The term hypnoanalgesia is mainly restricted to the pain insensitivity induced in such acute settings. While the mainstay of chronic pain treatment is the same set of techniques that are used in the treatment of anxiety, the specific hypnoanalgesic techniques may be co-opted from acute care. These specific techniques may provide some relief in problematic cases and provide some refreshing variation in clinical practice.

The term hypnoanalgesia will be avoided here, as similar effects can be obtained in relaxed states other than hypnosis. An early specific relaxation/hypnosis pain reduction method commences with the creation of local numbness/analgesia in the hand. The relaxed patient is asked to create the experience of having a hand in a bucket of ice water and to produce a feeling of coldness progressing to numbness or deadness. The hand may then be moved to a particular site, and the patient is asked to experience the numbness of the hand passing to the second site. This method is complicated, involving a number of steps, any of which may be a source of difficulty, and is not recommended. It was perhaps popular because the passing of analgesia from one region to another was spectacular and held some entertainment value. It is included here because it has historical value and gives us an idea of the possibilities.

An alternative method is to ask the patient

to create the experience of numbness as it occurs with the injection of local anaesthetic. To assist in the creation of the effect the patient can be asked first to experience the prick of a needle and then a sting as if a bolus had been injected, and finally a slowly spreading numbness. This numbness can be produced at any site, and the technique can be used to supplement the pain relief of general relaxation.

Another technique that has been used in the management of acute pain (burns dressing, surgery, dental work) is 'projection of the body image' to a distant location. The patient is asked to create the experience of the body part (or even the whole body) floating away to a distant place. In preparatory discussion, the therapist and patient agree that if a particular piece of anatomy is at a distant location, it cannot be 'here' and thus cannot be painful. Whether this mechanistic explanation is necessary is doubtful; as has been mentioned, any task that requires focused attention has the ability to reduce the experience of pain.

Visualizing a scene has been described above as a means of inducing relaxation. It is also reported to be useful in acute pain situations, under the designation, 'reduction of awareness by distraction'. We are not usually aware of the touch of our clothes; thus, if we are distracted, we may not be fully aware of nociceptive stimuli. The more able the patient is to focus and the greater detail that can be experienced, the better will be the analgesic effect.

The lessons of Ainslie Meares (1968) are most useful in helping people with pain. He pointed out that pain is a warning sign that the body is being harmed, but it is when the patient becomes emotionally distressed that pain becomes aversive and excessive. 'Unless we react to it there is little or no hurt in the painful stimulus.' He makes the point that when a child falls and is distressed, mother's kisses on the cheek markedly reduce the crying. Her kisses (to the cheek, not the knee) ease the emotional distress, not the nociceptive focus. Thus Meares points to the need for the patient to understand the nature of pain and to be confident that when emotional distress can be controlled (by relaxation) there is no need to be, or possibility of being overwhelmed, by pain.

Meares (1968) described a range of reactions to pain, including depression and hostility. In keeping with his insight that the amount of hurt associated with pain is proportional to the associated emotional distress, he recommends that patients are helped to a philosophical response. 'It can't be helped, but I will get over it.' Relaxation exercises can assist in shaping this response.

Finally, Meares (1968) acknowledges the possibility of pain relief by the above-mentioned methods, but favours the 'feeling of pain in its pure form'. He supplies us with the knowledge that pain is a signal; and, in a state of relaxation, the patient is able to experience pain as information rather than as an unbearable sensation.

Script 3

This monologue demonstrates a means of rapidly achieving relaxation. It is appropriate for the patient who has had some earlier lessons. It includes instructions on creating local analgesia.

Please close your eyes and follow my suggestions to the best of your ability . . . Let your legs relax . . . Let your back relax . . . Let your face relax . . . Let your whole body become pleasantly heavy and relaxed . . . Let your shoulders and arms relax . . . Let your neck relax . . . Now you are almost completely relaxed . . . Now you can slow your breathing . . . Let your feet relax . . . Let your hands relax . . . I am going to stop talking for a minute . . . Think about every part of your body in turn . . . you are a detective . . . check every part . . . make sure it is relaxed . . . If you find a part that is still tense . . . relax it as you breathe out . . . Move your index finger when you are fully relaxed.

Great . . . You are relaxed and calm . . . Feel calm . . . Feel calm all over . . . Let the feeling of calm float around you and through you . . . I will stop talking and let you focus on being calm . . . deeply relaxed and calm.

Now think of where your pain is . . . Try to imagine a local injection where your pain is . . . Feel a prick and a sting as the injection goes in . . . Calm and heavy . . . Calm and heavy . . . Now feel that area going numb . . . Feel numbness spreading out . . . dulling your pain . . . Let your pain become dull . . . Make your pain dull . . . Make that area numb and your pain dull . . . I will let you focus on making that area numb and your pain dull.

OK. Time to start coming back . . . You are relaxed and feeling good . . . You have lessened your pain . . . You have been able to take charge . . . Try to keep your pain area numb . . . Getting lighter . . . Still in charge . . . Getting lighter . . . OK . . . You can open your eyes whenever you want . . . You are still in control.

Script 4

This monologue demonstrates a very quick method of inducing deep relaxation. This is only appropriate for patients who have learned the basic skill of relaxation. The monologue also guides visualization of a beach scene and ends with the patient's accepting the pain as a nuisance, but something that can be tolerated.

Please close your eyes and relax . . . I am going to count to five . . . I want you to relax as I count . . . Five is very deeply relaxed . . . One is where you are now . . . just sitting quietly with your eyes closed . . . OK, getting ready . . . Starting at one, now relax down to two . . . Feeling relaxed . . . Going down now to three . . . Now you are moderately relaxed . . . Heavy in your chair . . . Slow your breathing . . . Get ready and now down to four . . . Now you are deeply relaxed . . . Calm and relaxed . . . Heavy and relaxed . . . Get ready and now come down to five . . . very deeply relaxed . . . I will give you a minute to make the last step down.

That's good . . . You are able to control your mind and body . . . Now try to imagine sitting or lying at the beach . . . Calm and relaxed . . . take your time and see the blue of the water and the sky . . . Calm and relaxed . . . waiting to be able to see the water and the sky . . . Are there any clouds in the sky? . . . If there are some clouds . . . move the index finger of your left hand . . . If there are no clouds, move the index finger of your right hand.

OK, there are some clouds . . . Now see the sand . . . focus on the sand . . . Try to see some seaweed on the sand . . . You are doing well . . . Deeply relaxed . . . Now try to feel the sun on your face . . . try to feel the warmth on your face . . . concentrate on the feeling of the sun on your face.

Now, think about your pain . . . Stay calm and relaxed . . . Your pain is a message . . . Your pain is a message you don't need . . . Stay calm and relaxed . . . Accept your pain as a nuisance . . . Something you don't need . . . But something you can live with . . . You are

in control . . . You are calm and feeling good . . . You are feeling fine . . . in spite of your pain . . . Calm and peaceful . . . You can accept your pain . . . You are doing well . . . Stay feeling calm . . . Now gradually come back up . . . and open your eyes.

The problem of non-compliance

Most patients are able to obtain some relief from anxiety and chronic pain through relaxation, hypnosis or meditation. However, many do not persist with these techniques. This is surprising, given that the pain is ever present and other treatment options are problematic and offer little relief. While these techniques may have a modest temporary effect, they are endlessly repeatable.

The reasons why they are abandoned, why patients cease claiming these analgesic benefits, include the facts that the techniques are time-consuming, require effort and provide only partial relief. Further, chronic pain is distressing and exhausting, making effort more difficult. Finally, these techniques can be boring.

There is little awareness that patients with chronic pain often discontinue these techniques. Patients often do not offer this information because they have been 'sold' the techniques as solutions to the pain, and they therefore feel ungrateful and embarrassed about their discontinuation. Therapists often do not ask too closely, as they do not want to know that the techniques have been abandoned, because they have little else to offer.

Why are these techniques presented as being highly effective when clinically, more accurately, they are moderately effective? Part of the answer may be that they are purveyed by therapists who are strongly biased in this direction. Another part may be that if these techniques are presented/accepted as being highly effective, then continuing pain means failure of the patient to make use of the prescribed treatment. The problem (pain) then becomes the sole responsibility of the patient, and the therapist becomes an unappreciated healer.

As chronic pain is an area of limited treatment options, and relaxation, hypnosis and meditation techniques can provide moderate relief, it is important to ensure full utilization. The following may encourage long-term compliance:

1. Give realistic expectations.
2. Emphasize that every option must be fully utilized.
3. Emphasize the need for regular, indefinite practice.
4. Tell the patient that minimal benefits will be available initially, but that worthwhile benefits will be available after a few weeks of regular practice.
5. Create interpersonal relationships such that patients will speak openly about the difficulties they are having finding time and energy to continue.
6. Detect when the techniques have been discontinued. Be accepting, but encourage re-commencement.
7. Combat boredom by finding techniques that suit the patient, and provide a range of techniques.
8. Closely monitor progress and try to find solutions to obstructions.
9. Remember, nothing works for everyone, and these techniques are not a panacea. This does not mean that either the patient or the therapist has failed.
10. If patients have become non-compliant and return for treatment, it is not enough simply to encourage them to recommence their technique. It is usually necessary to teach the technique again. This may seem odd, but, as with the behavioural treatment of agoraphobia and other phobias, relapsed patients need re-education in something they have already been taught.

References

Ashton C, Whitworth G, Seldomridge J, Shapiro P, Weinberg A, Michler R, Smith C, Rose E, Fisher S, Oz M. Self-hypnosis reduces anxiety following coronary artery bypass surgery. A prospective trial. *Journal of Cardiovascular Surgery* 1997; 38: 69–75.

Fisher P, Durham R. Recovery rates in generalized anxiety disorder following psychological therapy: an analysis of clinically significant change in the STSI-T across outcome studies since 1990. *Psychological Medicine* 1999; 29: 1425–34.

Jacobson E. *Progressive Relaxation*. University of Chicago Press, Chicago, 1938.

Kaplan K, Goldenberg D, Galvin-Nadeau M. The impact of a meditation-based stress reduction program on fibromyalgia. *General Hospital Psychiatry* 1993; 15: 284–9.

Lang E, Benotsch E, Fick L, Lutgendorf S, Berbaum M, Berbaum K, Logan H, Spiegel D. Adjunctive non-pharmacological analgesia for invasive medical procedures: a randomised trial. *Lancet* 2000; 355: 1486–90.

Lewis D. Hypnoanalgesia for chronic pain: the response to multiple inductions at one session and to separate single inductions. *Journal of the Royal Society of Medicine* 1992; 85: 620–4.

Meares A. *Relief without Drugs*. Souvenir Press, London, 1968.

Miller J, Fletcher K, Kabat-Zinn J. Three-year follow-up and clinical implications of a mindfulness meditation-based stress reduction intervention in the treatment of anxiety disorders. *General Hospital Psychiatry* 1995; 17: 192–200.

NIH Technology Assessment Panel on Integration of Behavioral and Relaxation Approaches into the Treatment of Chronic Pain and Insomnia. Integration of behavioral and relaxation approaches into the treatment of chronic pain and insomnia. *Journal of the American Medical Association* 1996; 276: 313–18.

Scott D. *Modern Medical Hypnosis*. Lloyd-Luke Ltd, London, 1974.

Stein C. The clenched fist technique as a hypnotic procedure in clinical psychotherapy. *American Journal of Clinical Hypnosis* 1963; 3: 113.

Wentworth-Rohr I. *Symptom reduction through clinical biofeedback*. Human Sciences Press Inc, New York, 1988.

Wilson P. *The Calm Technique*. Penguin Books, Ringwood, Australia, 1995.

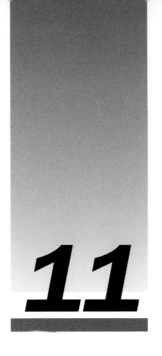

Psychotherapy in chronic pain

'... it has been consistently demonstrated by research that an alliance built on trust and, above all, a warm, non-judgmental and empathetic attitude in the therapist, lies at the heart of good therapy.'

Bloch and Singh, 1997

Reasonable proficiency in relaxation techniques can be developed through reading, attending short courses and regular use of techniques in clinical practice. Proficiency in psychotherapy, by contrast, requires extensive training and supervision. A chapter such as this can provide only preliminary information. Nevertheless, some useful principles are introduced.

Psychotherapy is defined (Sullivan, 1954) as primarily a verbal interchange between two individuals in which one of these is designated an expert and the other a help-seeker (for present purposes, a patient). They work together according to an established theory of personality, psychopathology and psychotherapy. They work together to identify the patient's characteristic problems in living, with the intention of achieving behavioural change. The potential behavioural change depends on the nature of the patient's symptoms, and the type and goals of psychotherapy, and may include shifts in understanding and attitude about the self and the world, symptom reduction, and in the now less common, most intense form, fundamental changes in personality.

While there are differences between various forms of psychotherapy, universal features have been identified (Frank, 1961), and include (1) a confiding relationship in which the therapist remains dependable, trustworthy and empathetic; (2) a rationale or agreed approach to therapy; (3) the provision of new information; (4) the gaining of hope by the patient; and (5) the experience of   . success and mastery. Psychotherapy may also be associated with arousal and expression of emotion. Finally, the therapist is a model from which the patient learns attitudes and behaviours. Such 'socially determined learning' (Bandura, 1977) is a feature of most human relationships.

The effectiveness of psychotherapy has been established (Shapiro and Shapiro, 1982). However, as with any other potent therapy, the patient's condition can also be made worse. Strupp et al (1978) found that 3–6% of patients are made worse. This outcome is possible only when patients are poorly selected and inadequately trained clinicians attempt ambitious therapy. Such therapy is clumsily and rigidly applied. However, no harm, only good can come from building an alliance with a trusted and empathetic therapist (Bloch and Singh, 1997).

An array of psychotherapies extends from deep lengthy psychoanalysis through to here-and-now brief therapy, and from client-centred therapy, in which nurturing empathy is a principal feature to cognitive therapy, which has thinking as the primary focus. Complete coverage is impossible; instead, some points that have relevance to the chronic pain patient will be mentioned.

The appropriate psychotherapy or psychotherapeutic elements in a given case depend on the nature of the pain and its origin, the premorbid personality and adjustment, the clinician's training and the overall management plan.

Psychoanalysis

Psychoanalysis is conducted in one-hour sessions, four or five times a week, usually for about five years. It is held that subjective experiences of childhood give rise to conflicts. These are usually conceptualized as involving sexual or aggressive wishes. They are frequently unconscious, and it is the work of psychoanalysis to bring them into awareness. Conflicts lead to anxiety, depression, somatic symptoms, social and sexual inhibitions, and difficulties in interpersonal relationships. Understanding them enables the patient to change maladaptive patterns of behaviour.

A central tool is the interpretation of transference. Transference involves the bringing to new relationships of unconscious attitudes, expectations and means of relating that were learnt in earlier relationships, particularly those of the first few years of life. During the process of psychoanalysis the patient attributes to the analyst the characteristics of one or more important persons from the past, and eventually begins to respond to him or her using unconscious attitudes and expectations from the past. Whenever evidence of transference emerges the analyst interprets or points out the presumed origin of this material. There are usually unconscious mechanisms within the patient that function to keep such conflicts and attitudes from consciousness. These serve a defensive, homeostatic role. Commonly the interpretation is rejected; in psychoanalytic terminology, the interpretation is met with resistance. The resistance may then be interpreted, or exposed, by the analyst. When the patient is able to accept an interpretation he or she is said to gain insight. Through serial insights the patient gains deep self-understanding and is able to develop new attitudes, expectations and means of relating.

Psychoanalysis in chronic pain

For a range of reasons, including the length and expense of training in psychoanalysis and the length and expense of this treatment for individual patients, this form of treatment is generally less available now than it was in the early to middle twentieth century.

Where pain is due to psychological factors, it can be conceptualized as arising from unconscious conflicts. For example, pain may be a means of keeping a conflict from the conscious mind, or a manner of dealing with the guilt attached to a particular conflict. In such circumstances, treatment using psychoanalytic techniques could be applied.

Where pain has some physical basis but psychological difficulties are hampering recovery, psychoanalysis may be employed to reduce anxiety or depression and to improve interpersonal functioning. In such cases improvement in pain and adjustment to residual pain are features of a general improvement in self-understanding, the sense of self-worth and coping skills.

Psychoanalytic theory may be useful in understanding patients in a range of circumstances. For example, we may be able to detect the conflict underlying pain of psychological origin, or to recognize transference issues, when a patient responds to helpful clinicians in an inappropriately aggressive manner, which appears to have origins in early life. Such understanding does not lead automatically to psychoanalytic treatment, owing to practical issues such as cost or the unsuitability of many patients (for example, patients need to have at least some ability to sustain effort and relationships). Nevertheless, such understanding better equips us to help such patients using alternative methods.

Psychoanalysis has provided a basis for a range of less time-consuming and less expensive forms of treatment. These are known by various names including psychoanalytic psychotherapy, 'dynamic psychotherapy' and 'brief' or 'focal psychotherapy'. Sessions may occur once or twice per week and, from the outset, be limited to less than twenty. In these, transference phenomena are neither encouraged nor extensively interpreted. The therapist is more active, and seeks to clarify and extend the patient's understanding in an empathetic setting.

Supportive psychotherapy

Two quite different categories of patient benefit from supportive psychotherapy. One is the patient who has a long history of coping poorly with the tasks of independent living. Such a person may find difficulty in reaching decisions, suffer feelings of low self-esteem, worry excessively about the opinions of others and claim inability to sustain effort. These patients may be unsuitable for change-orientated therapy such as psychoanalysis. The aim of supportive psychotherapy with such patients is to help them regain and maintain their best possible level of functioning, given their personality limitations and life circumstances. This is a form of long-term therapy.

The other type of patient who receives supportive psychotherapy is the individual who normally functions well in home, work and social settings, but has experienced extraordinary life events that have caused emotional distress and overwhelmed the ability to function independently. Here the focus is on regaining the former high level of functioning. Depending on the system of classification, instead of supportive psychotherapy, some would call this 'crisis intervention' therapy. With such individuals, change-orientated therapy is usually not indicated, and supportive psychotherapy is a short-term treatment.

The methods used include helping the individuals to understand their predicament, break complex tasks into manageable pieces, explore a range of solutions, and decide on a particular solution. Reassurance and encouragement are given as tasks are attempted. Patients are given information and advised toward realistic expectations. Empathy and even sympathy are important. There is a place for catharsis, which is the relatively unbridled expression of anxiety, depression, guilt, anger and the other distressing emotions that are stored up during a difficult life.

The risk in supportive psychotherapy is that the patient may become increasingly dependent on the therapist. This issue must be openly discussed; the patient should continue to use other supports and the therapist should ensure that the patient continues to take some decisions and actions as an independent individual. This issue is discussed in the early stages, and it is wise to place a time-limit on therapy. This may be a relatively long time, such as six months or one year. Then there should be a break in supportive psychotherapy, or at least a change of therapist; but a return is possible for a further series of sessions in the future.

Supportive psychotherapy is sometimes criticized because the aim is not progressive improvement in function. However, providing a 'holding environment', listening empathically and being a safe and reliable support may, in fact, lead to strengthening of the personality (Ornstein, 1986). Change also occurs through social learning (Bandura, 1977).

Supportive psychotherapy in chronic pain

Those people who have healthy personalities and have functioned well prior to an accident or injury that has resulted in chronic pain may benefit from supportive psychotherapy. Of course, chronic pain can mobilize previously contained conflicts, in such a way that dynamic psychotherapy may become appropriate.

For those patients who have pain of psychological origin or difficulty adjusting to chronic pain, but are unsuitable for dynamic psychotherapy, supportive psychotherapy may have a place. As was mentioned above, some individuals lack the necessary psychological skills and personality strengths to engage in change-orientated psychotherapy. With respect to chronic pain patients, two special cases deserve mention. Alexithymia, which means being 'without words to describe emotions' (Sifneos, 1996) is a personality feature that is reported to be an important factor in some cases of chronic pain. It is proposed that, in the absence of the ability to describe emotions, individuals respond to life situations in maladaptive ways, including the development of pain for which insufficient organic basis can be discovered. This inability to describe emotions and associated features such as a limited fantasy life make alexithymic individuals unsuitable for psychoanalytic-type therapy.

Contrary to the expectations of some, the presence of 'secondary gain' from a condition (including chronic pain) generally means the patient is unsuitable for change-orientated therapy. Where there are gains such as financial and emotional support, motivation for psychological change is limited. Change-orientated therapy calls for high levels of motivation. Thus chronic pain patients who are obtaining significant 'secondary gains' are usually better managed using supportive psychotherapy.

Cognitive therapy (CT) and cognitive behaviour therapy (CBT)

CT is usually a short-term treatment of 10 to 20 sessions, which are conducted once or, at most, twice per week. It is a system of psychotherapy that aims at symptom removal rather than resolution of underlying conflicts, as in psychoanalysis and the related psychotherapies. CT is based on the theory that characteristic 'errors in information processing' occur in depression, anxiety, personality disorder and other states of emotional distress (Wright and Beck, 1996).

These errors in information processing have also been called 'pathological information processing', 'cognitive distortions' and 'crooked thinking' (Ellis, 1962). They do not arise from organic pathology, as do the information processing or cognitive difficulties of dementia. Instead, these errors of information processing relevant to CT are more a matter of thinking style or habit. They occur in response to environmental stimuli. For example, if a person prone to depression makes a mistake at work, he or she might think, 'That just proves how dumb I am.' The person prone to anxiety, however, may avoid taking action, thinking, 'If I make a mistake they'll think I'm absolutely stupid.'

Central to CT theory is that errors in information processing result in emotional distress and maladaptive behaviour, rather

than the other way around (which may also be the case in certain circumstances). CT aims to correct errors in information processing as a means of relieving emotional distress. Therapists explore the thinking style and habits of patients and offer and encourage the use of logical perspectives and more adaptive responses. Where social withdrawal and other self-defeating behaviours have developed, behavioural modification is also encouraged: examples include relaxation exercises and assertiveness training.

CT does not claim that errors of information processing are the sole or even the initial causative feature of the syndromes of interest. The authors acknowledge the importance of genetics, early life experiences, interpersonal conflict and other factors known to have aetiological importance in mental disorders. Instead, CT is construed as a means of treatment of certain symptoms, and as a helpful technique that can be used in combination with medication (Simons et al, 1984).

CT is an expanding catalogue of techniques. Albert Ellis (1962), a pioneer in the field who coined the term 'rational emotive therapy' (RET), restricted his activities to disclosing 'crooked thinking' and teaching logical thinking. Later workers added behavioural techniques. Specific CT approaches have been developed for the treatment of depression (Beck et al, 1979), anxiety disorders (Beck et al, 1985), personality disorders (Beck et al, 1990) and other conditions.

Which particular techniques are included under the CT umbrella is largely a matter of personal opinion. With the addition of behavioural components, some have used the designation 'cognitive behaviour therapy' (CBT) for this form of psychotherapy. There is argument about the appropriateness of subsuming age-old techniques such as hypnosis and relaxation under the CT heading, as this could be taken incorrectly to suggest that the clinician needs special CT training to be qualified to deliver these services.

Cognitive therapy in chronic pain

All clinicians involved in the treatment of chronic pain provide accurate information to patients about the nature of chronic pain and encourage them to think logically and constructively about their situation. A particular example occurs when managing a person with pain-related fear who is inactive and becoming disabled because of the erroneous belief that pain indicates further structural damage. Appropriate interventions are consistent with the CT approach.

Current CT activities can be grouped under two main headings: cognitive restructuring and coping skills.

Cognitive restructuring is the correcting of errors in information processing. An example

of how this may apply in chronic pain is taken from Turner and Romano (1990): a patient who thinks 'I can't take this any more' is encouraged to more adaptive thinking, such as 'Is it really true that I can't deal with this? No. It may be difficult, but I've done it before and can again.'

Coping skills is a range of techniques including relaxation, hypnosis and meditation. 'Coping self-statements' may be placed under the general heading of coping skills, or enjoy a separate heading. Examples from Turner and Romano (1990) include: 'Relax', 'I can cope' and 'Focus on what you have to do.'

CT has much to offer in the management of the negative self-concepts and moods that may be associated with chronic pain and disability. CT and educational activities in general help patients make the best possible adjustments to their situations.

Summary

Psychotherapy is a vast theoretical and service landscape. Three points that represent different approaches have been described. All aim to reduce emotional distress. Psychoanalysis is a lengthy process that works to develop insight and resolution of unconscious conflicts, thereby reducing symptoms and encouraging growth of the personality. Supportive psychotherapy predominantly supports and encourages and thereby maintains the best possible functioning of severely impaired individuals. Cognitive therapy is a short-term psychotherapy that corrects errors in thinking style, thereby easing secondary emotional distress. It may also involve reversing maladaptive behaviour.

No psychotherapy has been expressly designed for application in chronic pain. However, they can all contribute to the general emotional well-being of chronic pain patients and favourably influence the experience of pain to some extent, depending on the personality and life circumstances of the individual and the nature of the pain.

Psychotherapy alone is rarely a satisfactory treatment of chronic pain (Pilowsky and Barrow, 1990), and this chapter does not pretend to teach psychotherapy. However, psychotherapy provides useful advice about the productive patient–clinician relationship and central elements of therapy. The psychotherapeutic relationship is confiding and empathetic. The patient and clinician agree on the therapeutic approach, exchange information and ensure that each understands the other. Hope and the trial of new or regained skills are encouraged, attempts are acknowledged. The therapist is a model and the therapist's attitudes, beliefs and behaviour are learned by the patient.

References

Bandura A. *Social Learning Theory*. Prentice-Hall, Englewood Cliffs, NJ, 1977.

Beck A, Rush A, Shaw B, et al. *Cognitive Therapy of Depression*. Guilford, New York, 1979.

Beck A, Emery G, Greenberg R. *Anxiety Disorders and Phobias: A Cognitive Perspective*. Basic Books, New York, 1985.

Beck A, Freeman A, et al. *Cognitive Therapy of Personality Disorder*. Guilford, New York, 1990.

Bloch S, Singh B. *Understanding Troubled Minds*. Melbourne University Press, Melbourne, 1997; 296.

Ellis A. *Reason and Emotion in Psychotherapy*. Lyle Stuart, New York, 1962.

Frank J. *Persuasion and Healing*. Williams and Wilkins, Baltimore, MD, 1961.

Ornstein A. Supportive psychotherapy: a contemporary view. *Clinical Social Work Journal* 1986; 14: 14–30.

Pilowsky I, Barrow C. A controlled study of psychotherapy and amitriptyline used individually and in combination in the treatment of chronic intractable, 'psychogenic' pain. *Pain* 1990; 40: 3–19.

Shapiro D, Shapiro D. Meta-analysis of comparative therapy outcome studies: a replication and refinement. *Psychological Bulletin* 1982; 92: 581–604.

Sifneos P. Alexithymia: past and present. *American Journal of Psychiatry* 1996; 153 (7 Suppl): 137–42.

Simons A, Garfield S, Murphy G. The process of change in cognitive therapy and psychopharmacology for depression: sustained improvement over one year. *Archives of General Psychiatry* 1984; 41: 45–51.

Strupp H, Hadley S, Gomes-Schwartz B. *Psychotherapy for Better or for Worse: The Problem of Negative Effects.* J Aronson, New York, 1978.

Sullivan H. *The Psychiatric Interview.* In: Perry H, Gawel M (eds) WW Norton, New York, 1954.

Turner J, Romano J. Cognitive-Behavioral Therapy. In: Bonica J (ed) *The Management of Pain* Lea and Febiger, Philadelphia, 1990.

Wright J, Beck A. Cognitive Therapy. In: Hales R, Yudofsky S (eds) *The American Psychiatric Press Synopsis of Psychiatry.* American Psychiatric Press, Washington, DC, 1996; 991–1010.

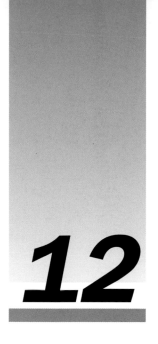

Fibromyalgia

'Merely corroborative detail, intended to give artistic verisimilitude to an otherwise bald and unconvincing narrative.'

WS Gilbert (The Mikado)

Introduction

Fibromyalgia (FM) is at the severe end of the spectrum of widespread pain. With broad diagnostic criteria, widespread pain was observed in 11.2% of a section of the British population (Croft et al, 1993). Fibromyalgia has been observed in 2% of a section of the North American population (Wolfe et al, 1995; Lawrence et al, 1998).

FM (and its forerunner, fibrositis) has been a contentious condition. Some authorities view the condition as a variant of anxiety, and point out that panic disorder was, for many decades, considered to be a heart condition (Skerritt, 1983). However, The American College of Rheumatology adopted diagnostic criteria in 1990 (Wolfe et al, 1990). These include widespread pain (defined as pain in the left and right sides of the body as well as above and below the waist), for at least 3 months. Axial pain (defined as pain in the cervical spine, anterior chest, thoracic spine or low back) must be present. In addition, the patient must report pain in at least 11 of 18 designated sites on digital palpation. While there may be problems with these criteria in so far as they are restrictive, they have allowed standardization of research.

Additional, commonly occurring symptoms/conditions, which are however not diagnostic criteria, include fatigue and non-restorative sleep, irritable bowel syndrome (IBS), Raynaud's syndrome-like symptoms, headache, subjective swelling, paraesthesia, palpitations, significant functional disability, psychological distress (including depression or anxiety) and cognitive complaints (particularly memory problems and inability to concentrate).

The aetiology of FM is unknown. Several mechanisms may be involved. A high prevalence in the female relatives of FM patients suggests a genetic vulnerability (Buskila & Neumann, 1997). In the related condition of somatization, genetic factors accounted for 25–50% of the total variance in reports of symptoms, whereas familial and environmental effects accounted for virtually no variance (Kendler et al, 1995). Onset often appears to follow physical or psychological stress. The majority (70%) of patients identify both physical and psychosocial factors (Neerinckx et al, 2000). Compared to healthy individuals, there is evidence that those with FM have suffered more stressful events in early life and in the previous year (Anderberg et al, 2000a); this does not, however, resolve questions of cause and effect.

The prognosis is poor. At 3-year follow-up, only 3% of patients were found to be free of all pain (Felson and Goldenberg, 1986). Current treatment is far from satisfactory.

FM is commonly associated with psychiatric disorders. Macfarlane et al (1999) found that over 25% of those with generalized pain (not precisely FM) had some concomitant mental disorder, most commonly depression. Anderberg et al (1999) found higher figures for FM: 37% suffering depression and 16% suffering anxiety. Depression in FM is independent of the cardinal features of pain severity and hypersensitivity to pressure pain (Okifuji et al, 2000); however, it may contribute to the inability fully to perform the activities of daily life.

FM patients tend to feature high levels of harm avoidance (Anderberg et al, 1999) and a strong tendency to catastrophizing (Hassett et al, 2000). There is evidence that unexplained physical symptoms (which include FM) are associated with abnormal attachment style (Taylor et al, 2000). This suggests that patients with poorer relationships will have poorer social and emotional supports and are more likely to present with such symptoms to the doctor.

Overlap

There is discussion about symptom overlap between FM and chronic fatigue syndrome (CFS), temporo-mandibular joint disorder (TMD), somatoform disorder and other medically unexplained syndromes.

Some special interest groups want CFS to be accepted as separate condition. The evidence to decide this point is still being accumulated.

Clauw and Chrousos (1997) point out that CFS has severe chronic fatigue as a necessary diagnostic feature, which must occur in the presence of four of eight symptoms (myalgia, arthralgia, sore throat, tender nodes, cognitive difficulty, headache, post-exertional malaise, sleep disturbance), and that five of these are pain-based. FM, however, has pain as the single necessary and sufficient feature (albeit with particular conditions), and is frequently accompanied by fatigue, sleep disorder, cognitive difficulties, headache, post-exertional malaise and sleep disturbance.

In a recent study 58% of females and 80% of males with fibromyalgia met the full criteria for CFS (White et al, 2000). Thus significant overlap between FM and CFS would seem to be beyond question.

Also, FM and CFS have similar comorbid illnesses/conditions, including IBS, interstitial cystitis and generalized pain sensitivity. The lifetime rates of IBS are 77% in FM and 92% in CFS (Aaron et al, 2000).

Pathophysiology

While the aetiology of FM remains uncertain, a range of pathophysiological phenomena have been reported. Which (if any) are primary and which are epiphenomena remains to be determined.

Naturally, the early studies focused on the structure of muscle. Fibres were sometimes described as 'moth-eaten' or in similar terms. However, such changes have not been observed in controlled studies, and FM is no longer considered to be a muscular disorder (Sims, 1998).

The pain threshold of peripheral structures and viscera is globally diminished. Parallel phenomena have been demonstrated for pressure, heat, cold and electrical stimulation (Dessein et al, 2000). These observations, in the absence of detectable peripheral pathology, have moved attention to the central nervous system.

Somatosensory-induced electroencephalographic potentials in FM are significantly different from those of normal individuals, and objectify the subjective reports of patients, indicating a lower pain threshold. There is a significant amplitude enhancement of cerebral potentials in response to painful CO_2-laser stimulation (Gibson et al, 1994; Lorenz et al, 1996).

Transcranial magnetic stimulation (TMS) was applied to the motor cortex of FM patients in various conditions (e.g. single pulse, paired pulse, relaxed and contracted muscles) (Salerno et al, 2000). Responses were captured from different sites and a range of calculations were performed. Motor cortical dysfunction was demonstrated in both excitatory and inhibitory mechanisms. However, similar findings were obtained from rheumatoid arthritis patients, and they may be a universal feature of chronic pain disorders.

The autonomic system is impaired. The sympathetic system may manifest diminished baseline tone, lability and a reduced responsiveness to stressors. Raj et al (2000) studied the heart rate over 24-hour periods and during tilt-table experiments. Qiao et al (1991) studied the conductance and blood flow of palmar skin during acoustic stimulation and cold pressor tests. The results of these studies suggest increased activity of cholinergic and decreased activity of adrenergic components of the peripheral sympathetic nervous system.

Non-restorative sleep is reported by 75% of FM patients (Wolfe, 1989). There is a well-established alpha wave intrusion during the non-REM sleep stages 3 and 4 (Moldofsky et al, 1975).

Endocrine abnormalities have been detected in hypothalamic–pituitary–adrenal axis (HPA) function, in low levels of growth hormone (GH) and insulin-like growth factor-1 (IGF-1 which is produced in response to GH and has many biological activities), in varying degrees of gonadal hypofunction, and

in blunted secretion of thyrotropin and thyroid hormone release in response to thyroid-releasing hormone (TRH) (Clauw and Chrousos, 1997).

On examining the HPA axis, the 24-hour levels of free cortisol in urine are low and there is a blunted cortisol response to exogenous CRH (Crofford et al, 1994). It may be relevant that 24-hour levels of free cortisol in urine are also significantly lower in CFS than in normal controls (Cleare et al, 2001). Returning to fibromyalgia, insulin-induced hypoglycaemia has been reported to both increase (Griep et al, 1993) and decrease (Alder et al, 1999) adrenocorticotropic hormone (ACTH) release. Very low levels of IGF-1 occur in one-third of FM patients, and may be specific to FM (Bennett et al, 1992).

The immune responses are frequently abnormal. Low natural killer cell numbers and function have been reported (Caro et al, 1993). However, the enhanced humoral immune responses that have been demonstrated in CFS do not appear to be a feature of FM.

Alterations in neurotransmitters and receptors are reported. The cerebrospinal fluid (CSF) has a threefold increase in substance P (SP: Vaeroy et al, 1988) and decrease in norepinephrine (NE: Russell et al, 1992a). Serum serotonin and tryptophan are decreased and the density of serotonin receptors on circulating platelets is increased (Russell et al, 1992b).

There is evidence of decreased regional cerebral blood flow in women with fibromyalgia. Comparing FM with healthy women, Montz et al (1995) found that those with FM demonstrated significantly lower regional cerebral blood flow (rCBF) of the cortex and thalamic and caudate nuclei. While this was a small study and replication is awaited, it points toward central changes in FM.

Speculation

As has been mentioned, which (if any) of the pathophysiological findings listed above are primary and which are epiphenomena remains to be determined. Nor is it always clear in which direction the biological events are occurring. Nevertheless, attempts have been made to organize the existing information.

FM as a sleep disorder

The hypothesis that FM is the result of sleep disorder is suggested by the frequent clinical finding of disturbed and non-restorative sleep, and fatigue. It is supported by the findings of alpha wave intrusion during the non-REM sleep stages 3 and 4 (Moldofsky et al, 1975) and the observation that disrupting the non-REM sleep of normal subjects leads to muscular aching and generalized tender points (Moldofsky and Scarisbrick, 1976). However, temazepam, melatonin and other hypnotics have been found to improve the sleep disorder without concomitant improvement in pain or fatigue.

Sleep has not been extensively studied in FM, and it remains unclear whether sleep disorder is a cause or consequence of the condition. However, important pieces of the puzzle include the facts that (1) low ILGF-1 levels may be related to sleep pathology, as GH secretion occurs during stage 4 sleep (Clauw and Chrousos, 1997), and (2) serotonin modulates stage 4 sleep (Moldofsky, 1982).

FM as a consequence of CNS sensitization

The pain threshold of a range of modalities is lower in FM than in normal controls. This has been objectified using evoked potentials. This leads, as no abnormality with muscle has been detected, to speculation regarding altered CNS sensory information processing. The term 'sensitization' is used in such circumstances, and is defined as an increased excitability of spinal and supraspinal neural circuits.

Sensitization develops consequent to ongoing nociceptive input. Various forms have been identified. One involves wide dynamic range (WDR) neurones; these are second-order dorsal horn neurones that respond to either non-nociceptive or nociceptive input. When WDR neurones become sensitized, consequent upon ongoing nociceptive input, they respond to all input, including non-nociceptive, as though it is nociceptive. Thus light touch or movement may cause pain (Gracely et al, 1992).

Once central sensitization has occurred, this mechanism could sustain painful muscles. It is possible that associated painful organ-specific syndromes such as IBS have a similar basis. As to the initiating event, FM is often consequent upon insults such as rheumatoid arthritis and osteoarthritis and physical trauma (it may also have roots in psychological trauma).

As has already been noted, in FM, the CSF SP may be three times the normal. This is important, as SP is believed to be a major factor in the process of central sensitization (Watkins et al, 1994).

FM as dysregulation of the stress response

This model posits that FM is a consequence of dysregulation of the human stress response, which is mediated predominantly by the endocrine and sympathetic systems. It has been argued that while the stress response was adaptive during human evolution, it is generally maladaptive for man in modern society, who rarely faces threats to survival (Meaney et al, 1993).

Mention has been made of reported impairments of the autonomic and endocrine systems in FM. A large number of reviews support the stress response dysregulation hypothesis (Clauw and Chrousos, 1997; Dessein et al, 2000; Heim et al, 2000; Neek, 2000; Neek and Croford, 2000; Torpy et al, 2000).

Corticotropin-releasing hormone (CRH) is a principal modulator in the stress response. The CRH neurones, which are mainly localized in the paraventricular nucleus of the hypothalamus, are widely distributed throughout the CNS. CRH has a profound effect on the function of the endocrine system. It also mediates arousal and stress-induced analgesia via beta-endorphin and excitatory amino acid-secreting neurones that project from the hypothalamus to the brain stem and spinal cord. It has input to the sympathetic system, which exerts antinociception via the spinal descending inhibitory pathways with the release of noradrenaline, serotonin and neuropeptide Y at the dorsal horn.

Thus the biological consequences of low CRH state are the opposite of that seen in acute stress and are similar to those noted in fibromyalgia and fatigue states: hypoarousal or fatigue and diffusely increased peripheral and visceral nociception (generalized pain). Also, along with the dysregulation of the autonomic system may come dysregulation of smooth muscle and cardiovascular function, which underpin at least some of the organ-specific syndromes (IBS, palpitations, Raynaud) that occur in this spectrum of disorders.

Various stressors can initiate the stress response. It is purported that continuous stress can cause the hypofunction and blunting of this response. The pain of FM is a stressor, and may become involved in a pathological self-sustaining cycle. It is proposed that CRH hyperactivity leads, eventually, to alteration of the set points of the various hormonal axes. Thus the observed hormonal deviations in FM may represent a CNS adjustment to chronic pain and stress.

Much attention in FM research has focused on the effect of CRH on the HPA axis. However, CRH also stimulates somatostatin secretion at the hypothalamic level, which in turn modulates GH secretion. (GH and IGF-1 levels have been reported as low in FM.) Daily GH injections given to a subgroup of FM patients with low serum IGF-1 levels produced a good response in 68% of subjects (Bennett et al, 1992). Thus dysregulation of the stress response may also influence GH levels.

As has been mentioned, serum serotonin has been reported as low. Serotonin can stimulate HPA axis activity. It is therefore possible that FM reflects a disorder of serotonin concentration or function. Alternatively, SP, which has been found elevated in CSF in FM, may have a role in inhibiting CRH secretion.

Speculation – summary

FM may prove to be a range of disorders with separate pathophysiologies. All of the above speculations have at least some underpinning that has been replicated. How to integrate this material is currently uncertain, but the final answer needs to address the following:

The evidence supporting FM as a primary sleep disorder is not strong, but symptomatic fatigue and sleep problems and the non-REM sleep abnormalities require explanation. The observed low ILGF-1 levels may be related to sleep pathology, as GH secretion occurs during non-REM sleep.

The evidence supporting a reduced pain threshold and a CNS sensitization is strong. This may be the result of various stressors. SP is elevated in CSF, and this may play a role in the sensitization process.

The evidence supporting dysregulation of the stress response system is moderately strong. There is evidence for some changes in endocrine and sympathetic systems function, but there is little to indicate whether this is cause or consequence. Dysregulation could logically follow sustained stress and could explain the generalized pain, the reduced arousal and some organ-specific syndromes.

The dysregulation of the stress response mechanisms is compatible with sensitization of the nervous system, and these two may be different faces of the same process. Abnormal GH level is a component of both the stress response dysregulation and the sleep disturbance, and may serve to integrate these hypotheses.

Serotonin in serum and SP in CSF may both be abnormal in FM. Both of these agents can influence the endocrine system function and play a role in CNS sensitization. Thus a neurotransmitter hypothesis may warrant consideration in the future.

Treatment

The response to treatment is poor. Most patients have used over-the-counter analgesics and a range of alternative treatments, such as vitamins and prayer. Many have also used acupuncture (which is now being incorporated into mainstream medicine) with some benefit (Berman et al, 1999).

In this setting of relative therapeutic impotence, it is especially important to attend to any concomitant psychiatric disorders. These can be anticipated in at least one-quarter of FM patients, and respond to standard treatments.

Exercise, education and CBT

Exercise, education and CBT have the advantage of being relatively free of side-effects and involving the patients in the treatment process. There is some evidence of efficacy, but less of prolonged benefit. Many treatment programmes include combinations of relaxation, meditation, cognitive restructuring, aerobic exercise and stretching, activity pacing and patient and family education. It is difficult for the clinician to determine which of these elements is or are responsible for any improvement.

Exercise programmes have produced significant reductions in pain and tender point count (Martin et al, 1996). Sleep and level of fatigue are unaffected. Long-term benefits, however, have not been demonstrated. In spite of the initial improvement, patients have ceased to exercise (Wigers et al, 1996).

Courses of cognitive behaviour therapy that aim to reduce the use of unhelpful behaviours such as excessive rest and over-monitoring of bodily symptoms and unhelpful attributions, and to increase confidence in the ability to manage symptoms, and that teach relaxation techniques, have produced promising results (Goldenberg et al, 1992). Unfortunately, long-term benefits have not been proved (Richards and Cleare, 2000).

Goossens et al (1996) compared the outcome of three treatment streams: (1) educational; (2) education plus cognitive therapy; and (3) the waiting list. Both treatment groups provided benefits. However, there was no significant difference in outcomes between the treatment groups. The addition of a cognitive component to the educational intervention led to significantly higher health-care costs, but no additional clinical benefit.

Antidepressants

In a relatively bare armoury, the tricyclic antidepressants, while only partially effective, are widely used. Arnold et al (2000) performed a meta-analysis of nine randomized controlled trials and found significant clinical response in 25–37% of patients. The largest improvements were in sleep quality, with other improvements in pain, stiffness, tenderness and fatigue. None of the studies that were examined used the dose ranges that are used in the treatment of depression; rather, the range was from 25 mg of amitriptyline to 75 mg of chlomipramine per day.

O'Malley et al (1999) conducted a meta-analysis of 94 placebo-controlled studies of antidepressants for unexplained symptoms and syndromes, 50 of which dealt with fibromyalgia. A majority (69%) demonstrated benefit for at least one outcome measure, and there was substantial benefit from medication. The absolute percentage difference in improvement between the antidepressant and placebo arms was 32%, yielding the conclusion that there would be a need to treat three persons for every person whose symptoms might be relieved.

While the tricyclic antidepressants are useful, the selective serotonin reuptake inhibitors (SSRIs) have been disappointing in treating the broad range of symptoms of fibromyalgia (O'Malley et al, 1999; Arnold et al, 2000). However, there is some evidence that they may be of value in the treatment of concurrent depression (Anderberg et al, 2000b).

Analgesics

Non-steroidal anti-inflammatory drugs (NSAIDs) have been disappointing. Ibuprofen was found to be no better, and naproxen only marginally better, than placebo (Richards and Cleare, 2000).

Bennett (1999) makes the statement: 'Currently opiates are the most effective medications for managing most chronic pain states.' However, opioids have not been extensively evaluated in fibromyalgia and receive little support in reviews (Millea and Holloway, 2000).

Tramadol is an analgesic with weak opioid and monaminergic actions. It has minimal respiratory depression, dependence and tolerance, and is more appropriate for long-term regular treatment than other forms of analgesia (Richards and Cleare, 2000). Leventhal (1999) suggested 'that tramadol may be useful for treatment of fibromyalgia pain'. This was followed by a group of letters that cautioned that this statement was premature and that side-effects limited usefulness. Biasi et al (1998) conducted a double-blind placebo-controlled trial using injectable preparations and found greater pain relief, but without reduction in the number of tender points. Further studies are needed, but a clinical trial of the oral form of this drug in difficult cases can be justified.

Local anaesthetic injection and dry needling

Injection of tender points with local anaesthetic is used in the effort to provide pain relief. Lignocaine has also been combined with triamcinolone. Piercing a tender point with a needle but injecting nothing (dry needling) may also be of benefit, suggesting that the release of met-enkephalin may be an important factor (Figuerola et al, 1998). These procedures require further examination, but are unlikely to cause damage.

Hormones

Oral corticosteroids have not been useful.

Bennett et al (1992) found that in the subgroup of patients with low IGF-1, daily injections of GH produced a good global response in 68% of patients. This was not without side-effects: one-third of patients developed carpal tunnel syndrome. This is an expensive compound, and more work needs to be done before regular use could be considered.

Other treatments

Ondansetron, a selective 5HT3 receptor antagonist, has shown promise in a double-blind cross-over trial (Hrycaj et al, 1996). This is another expensive compound that may find a place in the treatment of FM in the future.

Ketamine, an N-methyl-D-aspartate (NMDA) receptor antagonist anaesthetic, given intravenously in sub-anaesthetic doses, has attenuated pain, increased pain threshold and improved muscle endurance in controlled trials (Sorensen et al, 1997). This agent has been associated with hallucinations, and further work is required.

There are many other drugs that have been found to have benefits in small studies that are awaiting replication.

References

Aaron L, Burke M, Buchwald D. Overlapping conditions among patients with chronic fatigue syndrome, fibromyalgia and termporomandibular disorder. *Archives of Internal Medicine* 2000; 164: 221–7.

Alder G, Kinsley B, Hurwitz S, Mossey C, Goldenberg D. Reduced hypothalamic–pituitary and sympathoadrenal responses to hyperglycemia in women with fibromyalgia syndrome. *American Journal of Medicine* 1999; 106: 534–43.

Anderberg U, Forsgren T, Ekselius L, Marteinsdottir I, Hallman J. Personality traits on the basis of the Temperament and Character Inventory in female fibromyalgia syndrome patients. *Nordic Journal of Psychiatry* 1999; 53: 353–9.

Anderberg U, Mareinsdottir I, Theorell T, von Knorring L. The impact of life events in female patients with fibromyalgia and in female healthy controls. *European Psychiatry* 2000a; 15; 295–301.

Anderberg U, Marteinsdottir I, von Knorring L. Citalopram in patients with fibromyalgia – a randomised, double-blind, placebo-controlled study. *European Journal of Pain* 2000b; 15: 295–301.

Arnold L, Keck P, Welge J. Antidepressant treatment of fibromyalgia. A meta-analysis and review. *Psychosomatics* 2000; 41: 104–13.

Bennett R. Emerging concepts in the neurobiology of chronic pain: evidence of abnormal sensory processing in fibromyalgia. *Mayo Clinic Proceedings* 1999; 74: 385–98.

Bennett R, Clark S, Campbell S, Burckhardt C. Low levels of somatomedin C in patients with fibromyalgia syndrome. *Arthritis and Rheumatism* 1992; 35: 1113–16.

Berman B, Ezzo J, Hadhazy V, Swyers J. Is acupuncture effective in the treatment of fibromyalgia? *Journal of Family Practice* 1999; 48: 213–18.

Biasi G, Manca S, Manganelli S, Marccolongo R. Tramadol in the fibromyalgia syndrome: a controlled clinical trial versus placebo. *International Journal of Pharmacological Research* 1998; 18: 13–19.

Buskila D, Neumann L. Fibromyalgia syndrome (FM) and nonarticular tenderness in relatives of patients with FM. *Journal of Rheumatology* 1997; 24: 941–4.

Caro X, Ojo-Amaize E. Agopian M, Peter J. Natural killer cell function in primary fibrositis (fibromyalgia) syndrome. *Arthritis and Rheumatism* 1993; 36(9S): D114.

Clauw D, Chrousos G. Chronic pain and fatigue syndromes: overlapping clinical and neuroendocrine features and potential pathogenic mechanisms. *Neuroimmunomodulation* 1997; 4: 134–53.

Cleare A, Blair D, Chambers S, Wessely S. Urinary free cortisol in chronic fatigue syndrome. *American Journal of Psychiatry* 2001; 158: 641–3.

Crofford L, Pillemer S, Kalogeras K, Cash J, Michelson D, Kling M et al. Hypothalamic–pituitary–adrenal axis perturbations in patients with fibromyalgia. *Arthritis and Rheumatism* 1994; 37: 1583–92.

Croft P, Rigby A, Boswell R, Schollum J, Silman A. The prevalence of chronic widespread pain in the general population. *Journal of Rheumatology* 1993; 20: 710–13.

Dessein P, Shipton E, Stanwix A, Joffe B. Neuroendocrine deficiency-mediated development and persistence of pain in fibromyalgia: a promising paradigm? *Pain* 2000; 86: 213–15.

Felson D, Goldenberg D. The natural history of fibromyalgia. *Arthritis and Rheumatism* 1986; 29: 1522–6.

Figuerola M, Loe W, Sormani M, Barontini M. Met-enkephalin increase in patients with fibromyalgia under local treatment. *Functional Neurology* 1998; 13: 291–5.

Gibson S, Littlejohn G, Gorman M, Heime R, Granges G. Altered heat and pain thresholds and cerebral event-related potentials following painful CO_2 laser stimulation in subjects with fibromyalgia syndrome. *Pain* 1994; 58: 185–93.

Goldenberg D, Kaplan K, Nadeau M. A prospective study of stress reduction, relaxation response therapy in fibromyalgia. *Scandinavian Journal of Rheumatology* 1992; S94: 47.

Goossens M, Rutten-van Molken M, Leidl R, Bos S, Vlaeyen J, Teeken-Gruben N. Cognitive-educational treatment of fibromyalgia: a randomised clinical trial. II. Economic evaluation. *Journal of Rheumatology* 1996; 23: 1246–54.

Gracely R, Lynch S, Bennett G. Painful neuropathy: altered central processing maintained dynamically by peripheral input (published erratum appears in *Pain* 1993; 52: 251–3). *Pain* 1992; 51: 175–94.

Griep E, Boersma J, de Kloet E. Altered reactivity of the hypothalamic–pituitary–adrenal axis in the primary fibromyalgia syndrome. *Journal of Rheumatology* 1993; 20: 469–74.

Hassett A, Cone J, Patella S, Sigal L. The role of catastrophizing in the pain and depression of women with fibromyalgia syndrome. *Arthritis and Rheumatism* 2000; 43: 2493–500.

Heim C, Ehlert U, Hellhammer D. The potential role of hypocortisolism in the pathophysiology of stress related bodily disorders. *Psychoneuroendocrinology* 2000; 25: 1–35.

Hrycaj P, Stratz T, Mennet P, Muller W. Pathogenic aspects of responsiveness to ondansetron (5HT type 3 receptor antagonist) in patients with primary fibromyalgia syndrome – a preliminary study. *Journal of Rheumatology* 1996; 23: 1418–23.

Kendler K, Walters E, Truett K, Heath A, Neale M, Martin N. A twin-family study of self-report symptoms of panic-phobia and somatization. *Behavior and Genetics* 1995; 25: 499–515.

Lawrence R, Helmick C, Arnett F, et al. Estimated prevalence of arthritis and selected musculoskeletal disorders in the United States. *Arthritis and Rheumatism* 1998; 41: 778–99.

Leventhal L. Management of fibromyalgia. *Annals of Internal Medicine* 1999; 131: 850–8.

Lorenz J, Grasedyck K, Bromm B. Middle and long latent somatosensory evoked potentials after painful laser stimulation in patients with fibromyalgia syndrome. *Electroencephalography and Clinical Neurophysiology* 1996; 1000: 165–8.

Macfarlane G, Morris S, Hunt I, Benjamin S et al. Chronic widespread pain in the community: the influence of psychological symptoms and mental disorders on healthcare seeking behaviour. *Journal of Rheumatology* 1999; 26: 413–19.

Martin L, Nutting A, Macintosh B, et al. An exercise program in the treatment of fibromyalgia. *Journal of Rheumatology* 1996; 23: 1050–3.

Meaney M, Bhatnagar S, Larocque S, McCormick C, et al. Individual differences in the hypothalamic–pituitary–adrenal stress response and the hypothalamic CRH system. *Annals of the New York Academy of Sciences* 1993; 697: 70–85.

Millea P, Holloway R. Treating fibromyalgia. *American Family Physician* 2000; 62: 1575–82, 1587.

Moldofsky H. Rheumatic pain modulation syndrome: the interrelationships between sleep, central nervous system serotonin, and pain. *Advances in Neurology* 1982; 33: 51–7.

Moldofsky H, Scarisbrick P. Induction of neurasthenic musculoskeletal pain syndrome by selective sleep stage deprivation. *Psychosomatic Medicine* 1976; 38: 35–44.

Moldofsky H, Scarisbrick P, England R, Smythe H. Musculoskeletal symptoms and non-REM sleep disturbance in patients with 'fibrositis syndrome' and healthy subjects. *Psychosomatic Medicine* 1975; 37: 341–51.

Montz J, Bradley L, Modell J, Alexander R, Trian-Alexander M, Aaron L, et al. Fibromyalgia in women. Abnormalities of regional cerebral blood flow in the caudate nucleus are associated with low pain threshold levels. *Arthritis and Rheumatism* 1995; 38: 926–38.

Neek G. Neuroendocrine and hormonal perturbations and relations to the serotonergic system in fibromyalgia patients. *Scandinavian Journal of Rheumatology* 2000; 29 (Suppl 113): 8–12.

Neek G, Crofford L. Neuroendocrine perturbations in fibromyalgia and chronic fatigue syndrome. *Rheumatic Diseases Clinics of North America* 2000; 26: 989–1002.

Neerinckx E, Van Houdenhove B, Lysens R, Vertommen H, Onghena P. Attributions in chronic fatigue syndrome and fibromyalgia syndrome in tertiary care. *Journal of Rheumatology* 2000; 27: 1051–5.

Okifuji A, Turk D, Sherman J. Evaluation of the relationship between depression and fibromyalgia syndrome: why aren't they all depressed? *Journal of Rheumatology* 2000; 27: 212–19.

O'Malley P, Jackson J, Santoro J, Tomkins G, Balden E, Krownke K. Antidepressant therapy for unexplained symptoms and symptom syndromes. *Journal of Family Practice* 1999; 48: 980–90.

Qiao Z, Vaeroy H, Morkrid L. Electrodermal and microcirculatory activity in patients with fibromyalgia during baseline, acoustic stimulation and cold pressor tests. *Journal of Rheumatology* 1991; 18: 1383–9.

Raj S, Broullard D, Simpson C, Hopman W, Abdollah H. Dysautonomia among patients with fibromyalgia: a non invasive assessment. *Journal of Rheumatology* 2000; 27: 2660–5.

Richards S, Cleare A. Treating fibromyalgia. *Rheumatology* 2000; 39: 343–6.

Russell I, Vaeroy H, Javors M, Nyberg F. Cerebrospinal fluid biogenic amine metabolites in fibromyalgia/fibrositis syndrome and rheumatoid arthritis. *Arthritis and Rheumatism* 1992a; 35: 550–6.

Russell I, Mickalek J, Vipraio G, Fletcher E, Javors M, Bowden C. Platelet 3H-imipramine uptake receptor density and serum serotonin levels in patients with fibromyalgia/fibrositis syndrome. *Journal of Rheumatology* 1992b; 19: 104–19.

Salerno A, Thomas E, Olive P, Boltman F, Picot M, Georgesco M. Motor cortical dysfunction disclosed by single and double magnetic stimulation in patients with fibromyalgia. *Clinical Neurophysiology* 2000; 111: 994–1001.

Sims R. Fibromyalgia is not a muscular disorder. *American Journal of Medical Science* 1998; 315: 346–50.

Skerritt P. Anxiety and the heart – a historical review. *Psychological Medicine* 1983; 12: 17–25.

Sorensen J, Bengtsson A, Backman E, Henriksson K, Eksellus L, Bengtsson M. Fibromyalgia – are there different mechanisms in the processing of pain? A double blind crossover comparison of analgesic drugs. *Journal of Rheumatology* 1997; 24: 1615–21.

Taylor R, Mann A, White N, Goldberg D. Attachment style in patients with unexplained physical symptoms. *Psychological Medicine* 2000; 30: 931–41.

Torpy D, Papanicolaou D, Lotsikas A, Wilder R, Chrousos G, Pillemer S. Responses of the sympathetic nervous system and the hypothalamic–pituitary–adrenal axis to interleukin-6: a pilot study in fibromyalgia. *Arthritis and Rheumatism* 2000; 43: 872–80.

Vaeroy H, Helle R, Forre O, Kass E, Terenius L. Elevated CSF levels of substance P and high incidence of Raynaud phenomenon in patients with fibromyalgia: new features of the diagnosis. *Pain* 1988; 32: 21–6.

Watkins L, Wlertelak E, Furness L, Maler S. Illness-induced hyperalgesia is mediated by spinal neuropeptides and excitatory amino acids. *Brain Research* 1994; 664: 17–24.

White K, Speechley M, Harth M, Ostbye T. Co-existence of chronic fatigue syndrome with fibromyalgia syndrome in the general population. A controlled study. *Scandinavian Journal of Rheumatology* 2000; 29: 44–51.

Wigers S, Stiles T, Vogel P. Effects of aerobic exercise versus stress management treatment in fibromyalgia. A 4.5 year prospective study. *Scandinavian Journal of Rheumatology* 1996; 25: 77–86.

Wolfe F. Fibromyalgia: the clinical syndrome. *Rheumatic Diseases Clinics of North America* 1989; 15: 1–18.

Wolfe F, Smythe H, Yunus M, Bennett R, et al.

The American College of Rheumatology 1990 criteria for the classification of fibromyalgia. *Arthritis and Rheumatism* 1990; 33: 160–72.

Wolfe F, Ross K, Anderson J, Russell I, Hebert L. The prevalence and characteristics of fibromyalgia in the general population. *Arthritis and Rheumatism* 1995; 38: 19–28.

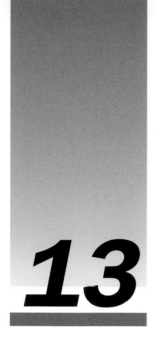

Headache

'The greater the ignorance the greater the dogmatism.'
Sir William Osler 1902

Headache is the most common pain disorder. In the USA the prevalence was 78% among adult women and 68% among adult males (Taylor 1985). In large community surveys, headache had occurred in the last 14 days in 19% (Rasmussen et al, 1991) and 21% (Wadsworth et al, 1971) of participants. Headache is more common in women than men (partly because of the higher prevalence in females of migraine and tension-type headache). This may be due to female hormones (Rasmussen, 1993). The prevalence decreases after middle age, and many subjects become symptom-free.

The impact on the individual varies from minimal, in the case of the individual with a mild occasional headache, through to profound in the case of severe, frequent migraine. Headache may cause considerable direct medical costs and incapacitate people during their most productive years.

Headache research and therapy is a sophisticated field of medicine. Comprehensive accounts are available (Olesen et al, 2000). This chapter only offers clinical suggestions for some major, recurrent categories of headache.

The Headache Classification Committee of the International Headache Society (IHS, 1988) produced a comprehensive classification of headache disorders, cranial neuralgias, and facial pain. Groups 1 to 4 are the primary headaches, which include migraine, tension-type headache and cluster headache, all of which receive attention in this chapter. Groups 5 to 11 are the secondary headaches. This grouping includes headache associated with disorders of the neck, which also receives mention later. Group 12 covers the cranial neurologias and facial pain, and Group 13 is concerned with 'headache not classifiable'; neither group receives further mention.

Migraine

Migraine is a familial disorder characterized by periodic, commonly unilateral, pulsatile headaches that begin in childhood, adolescence, or early adult life and recur with diminishing frequency during advancing years (Adams et al, 1997). It is common, occurring in 4–6% of men and 14–17% of women. The diagnosis depends on the history and the exclusion of other conditions.

Two forms are described (migraine without aura and migraine with aura). The advantage of this distinction is unclear, as the treatment is the same.

Diagnostic criteria for migraine without aura (IHS, 1988)

1. Attacks last 4–72 hours
2. At least two of:
   - unilateral
   - pulsating
   - moderate to severe
   - aggravated by movement.
3. At least one of:
   - nausea
   - photophobia
   - phonophobia.

Diagnostic criteria for migraine with aura (HIS, 1988)

1. At least three of:
   - one or more fully reversible aura symptoms occur, indicating brain dysfunction
   - at least one aura symptom develops gradually over more than 4 minutes, or two or more symptoms occur in succession
   - no single aura symptom lasts more than 60 minutes
   - headache follows aura with a free interval of less than 60 minutes (it may also begin before or simultaneously with the aura).
2. History, physical examination, and where appropriate, diagnostic tests exclude a secondary cause.

Aura

A subjective experience associated with (usually proceeding) the headache. Visual auras are by far the most common. These may occur in one or both eyes. The patient cannot see clearly to one side of the fixation point. This area of defective vision may be foggy or shimmering; zigzag lines suggesting the top of a castle (fortification or teichopsia) are common; coloured outlines and scotoma may occur.

Less common auras include paraesthesia, motor weakness and aphasias.

Auras may occur in combination.

Pathophysiology

The definitive pathophysiological explanation has not yet been achieved. Emotional stress and genetic factors may be important.

Vascular factors have been emphasized. Distension and excessive pulsation of branches of the external carotid artery has been speculated, and is supported by the observation that the throbbing quality of the headache may be relieved by compression of the parent artery (Iversen et al, 1990). Reduction of regional cerebral blood flow has been demonstrated during attacks (Leao, 1944).

A neural hypothesis suggests an abnormality in the trigeminal nerve and perhaps the hypothalamus (Lance, 1993).

Headache diary

A headache dairy is a means of keeping the patient involved in management and obtaining valuable information. It will establish a baseline and chart response to therapy. Details of dates (which give the frequency), severity, duration, auras, associated symptoms and suspected triggers (e.g. stress, menstruation, foods, caffeine withdrawal) should be recorded.

Non-drug therapy

A wide range of non-drug treatments, from relaxation exercises, psychotherapy and biofeedback to massage, chiropractic and homeopathy, have enthusiastic exponents. Some may have value by reducing 'stress'. Few have been examined in double-blind placebo-controlled trials. Medical practitioners should not obstruct the pursuit of non-drug therapy solutions; but where benefit is not obtained, they should discourage exploitation.

Opioids

Authoritative opinion is that opioids have little place in the treatment of migraine. They compound the delayed gastric emptying that is a feature of the disorder. Codeine and pethidine are short-acting, and recurrent headache (reappearance of a headache that had been significantly relieved) may occur.

Also there is the danger of drug dependence, particularly where control is difficult. Finally, there is evidence that these drugs, taken over time, may actually cause headache.

Pethidine, which is frequently sought and provided, has the additional disadvantage of having a metabolite (norpethidine) that is neurotoxic and a strong convulsant (Hassan et al, 2000).

Medication

Abortive (treatment of acute episodes) and prophylactic medication is available. Many medications are highly effective; the choice at any point depends on confounding medical conditions, past response, side-effects and cost. The aim in the following protocols is to provide safe, effective and, importantly, straightforward guidelines. Alternative, equally good, choices are possible.

Medical treatment of the acute episode

Commence treatment at the first sign. Withdraw to a quiet room with soft light and relax; if possible, sleep.

1. *Regimen One: Simple analgesic plus anti-emetic*
This regimen is suitable as the initial treatment for new patients, particularly when

the migraine is of mild or moderate severity. Like all migraine regimens, it is most effective when commenced early.

> Aspirin (900 mg) or paracetamol (1000 mg) plus metoclopramide (10 mg) or prochlorperazine (5 mg).

The analgesic can be repeated every 4 hours.

Points to remember:
a. Aspirin is contraindicated where there are enteric ulcers or bleeding disorders.
b. In pregnancy, prochlorperazine to be used up to 32 weeks, metoclopramide to be used after 32 weeks.
c. Give both the analgesic and the antiemetic, even if there is no nausea. Metoclopramide will speed gastric emptying.
d. Prochlorperazine has a mild sedative effect, which is often an advantage.
e. If vomiting is a concern, consider prochlorperazine 5 mg suppositories.
f. Prochlorperazine has been associated with acute dystonic reaction.
g. Both prochlorperazine and metoclopramide have been associated with akathisia – a distressing emotional and physical restlessness.
h. Treat acute dystonia and akathisia with an anticholinergic (e.g. benztropine 2 mg, orally or imi), followed after one hour, if

there is insufficient response, by diazepam 5 mg by mouth.

2. *Regimen Two: NSAID or 5-HT$_{1D}$ agonist plus antiemetic*

This regimen is appropriate as the routine treatment where the patient has, in the past, failed to achieve satisfactory results with Regimen One. It can also be implemented as a second-wave treatment if there is no sign of improvement with the application of Regimen One.

Naproxen (1000 mg, oral) or sumatriptan (50–100 mg, oral) plus an antiemetic, as above.

Naproxen can be repeated once, after 4 hours. Sumatriptan (50 mg) can be repeated after one hour; administration above 100 mg offers no additional benefit.

Points to remember:
a. Sumatriptan is contraindicated in pregnancy and where there are risk factors for cardiovascular or cerebrovascular accident.
b. Naproxen is contraindicated where there are enteric ulcers or bleeding disorders.
c. Sumatriptan is commenced with the onset of pain, not during the aura.
d. Sumatriptan (6 mg) is also available as a patient- or professional-administered subcutaneous injection. This can be repeated only once, after one hour, if there has been no improvement.
e. Naproxen (500 mg) is available as a suppository.

3. *Regimen Three: Antiemetic plus dopamine blockade*

This is appropriate treatment where Regimen One has failed and the doctor is able to provide a home visit.

Metoclopramide 10 mg imi plus chlorpromazine 50 mg orally or imi.

Points to remember:
a. In pregnancy, metoclopramide may be used only in the last trimester.
b. Chlorpromazine can be used throughout pregnancy and can be used alone in the first two trimesters. There is little point substituting prochlorperazine for metoclopramide in the first two trimesters, as prochlorperazine and chlorpromazine are from the same drug family (phenothiazines).
c. Metoclopramide is given by imi at this stage of the episode irrespective of vomiting. It reverses gastroparesis and reduces nausea.
d. Chlorpromazine given by imi is uncomfortable and may (rarely) lead to a sterile abscess. These are relatively low-priority issues at this stage of severe migraine. If vomiting is not a major

problem and metoclopramide has been administered, oral chlorpromazine may be considered.

e. Chlorpromazine will cause sedation, which will be an advantage.

f. Chlorpromazine may cause hypotension via an alpha-blocking action. Dizziness may be reported. This needs no specific therapy other than care with rising from sitting or lying and with walking.

g. Chlorpromazine theoretically can lead to acute dystonia and akathisia, but this is unlikely at this low dose. In such an event administer an anticholinergic and later, if necessary, a benzodiazepine, as outlined in Regimen One.

h. Ergotamines should not be administered within 24 hours of $5HT_{1D}$ agonists.

4. *Regimen Four: Lignocaine/lidocaine infusion*
This is appropriate for status migranosus (migraine lasting longer than three days), and hospital admission is indicated.

Lignocaine 2 mg/min delivered by pump. Duration not to exceed 14 days.

Points to remember:

a. Contraindications: significant cardiac disease, epileptic seizures, severe degrees of sinoatrial, atrioventricular or intraventricular heart block, or allergic reactions to lignocaine.

b. An ECG should be performed before and 60 minutes after commencement of infusion. Pulse rate, blood pressure and further ECGs to be performed according to local protocols.

Medical prophylaxis

A 50% reduction in headache frequency is a realistic goal of medical prophylaxis; fewer than 10% of patients achieve headache-free status.

Avoidance of triggers is the best prophylactic. But often there are no clear triggers, and in any case, avoidance may not give the desired degree of prophylaxis.

Most of the commonly used prophylactic agents produce a satisfactory response in about 60% of patients, and there is little evidence that one is superior to the rest. (A warning against undue confidence, however: the placebo response for most medical conditions is around 50%.) The choice of agent therefore depends on pre-existing medical conditions and adverse effects. With continuous administration there is greater probability of developing adverse effects. The adverse effects of each medication should be discussed so that the patient can be fully involved in selection.

1. *Beta-blocker*
Propranolol 40 to 300 mg per day or metoprolol 50 to 200 mg per day.
Start at low doses and increase gradually at two- to four-week intervals.

Points to remember:

a. Contraindications: congestive heart failure, atrioventricular conduction defects and peripheral vascular disease. They must be used with caution in diabetes, as they may mask some early signs of hypoglycaemia.

b. Propranolol is a non-selective beta-blocker, and is therefore contraindicated in patients with asthma. Metoprolol is a selective beta-1-blocker, and can be used with caution in patients with asthma.

c. Propranolol passes the blood–brain barrier, and depression is an important side-effect. Metoprolol passes the blood–brain barrier much less easily, and has not been associated with depression.

d. Other beta-blocker side-effects include fatigue, orthostatic hypotension, diarrhoea and insomnia.

e. Failure to respond to one beta-blocker does not predict failure to all; hence another selective drug with proven prophylactic efficacy, such as atenolol, could also be trialled.

f. Beta-blockers will not prevent the aura, but they can be used in migraine both with and without aura.

2. *Anticonvulsant*

Sodium valproate 800 to 2000 mg per day in divided doses.

Start at low dose (400 mg) and slowly titrate up to the plasma concentrations used in epilepsy. Beneficial effects may be achieved before reaching the anti-epileptic range.

Points to remember:

a. Contraindications: pregnancy, liver disease and thrombocytopenia.

b. Fulminant hepatitis is a serious but rare side-effect of these drugs, and is not consistently preceded by abnormal liver function tests.

c. Common adverse effects include nausea, weight gain, tremor and hair loss.

d. Baseline and regular full blood examination and liver function tests are recommended.

e. Gradual dose increases will reduce the likelihood of adverse effects.

3. *Tricyclic antidepressant (TCA)*

Amitriptyline 10 to 150 mg at night.

Commence at 10 mg at night and increase slowly. Some authorities limit the dose to 150 mg, but higher doses can be used, depending on tolerance of adverse effects.

Points to remember:

a. Contraindications: pregnancy, narrow-angle glaucoma and urinary retention.

b. Adverse effects: drowsiness, dry mouth, weight gain, orthostatic hypotension, constipation.

c. Dangerous in overdose.

d. Amitriptyline is the only TCA with established efficacy in migraine

prophylaxis. Imipramine and
clomipramine appear to be effective.

e. The anti-migraine effect is unrelated to
antidepressant effect.

f. To date, the SSRIs have not been shown
to be effective.

4. *NSAID*

Naproxen 500 mg twice daily

Points to remember:

a. Contraindications: peptic ulceration, liver
or kidney disease and coagulation
disorder/treatment.

b. Side-effects: erosive gastritis, diarrhoea,
fluid retention, haematological
complications.

d. For migraine associated with
menstruation: naproxen for one week
before through to one week after
menstruation.

e. Where erosive gastritis complicates
successful prophylaxis, consider combining
naproxen with a proton pump inhibitor
such as omeprazole 20 mg daily.

The patient and the doctor

In the management of migraine, the patient
and the doctor must work as a team. There
may also be other team players, including
family members, a psychologist, employers
and doctors from various fields.

The patient should keep a headache diary

and bring it to appointments. The doctor
should reassure, emphasize the importance of
early treatment and give information. They
should work together in the assessment of
response to non-medical treatment and to
acute and prophylactic medical treatment.
They should discuss the patient's daily routine
with a view to establishing regular sleep, and
explore psychosocial factors.

Tension-type headache

Tension headache is the most common form
of headache. It is more common in females,
and onset may be in middle life. Chronic
anxiety or depression is frequently present.

Tension headache is usually bilateral, but
may occur on one side. It does not always
occur in the same location. In order of
frequency it occurs in occipital, parietal,
temporal and frontal regions. It is described as
dull, aching, full or tight; often as if the head
were encircled by a tight band. There may be
throbbing. Sleep is usually not disturbed, but
the headache may be noticed soon after
waking. There may be grinding of the teeth
and tenderness around the head.

A thorough history and physical (including
neurological) examination is mandatory. The
aim is not only to exclude other diagnoses, but
to confirm the diagnosis of tension-type
headache. In the physical examination a
manual examination of pericranial muscles
may identify tender points (manual pressure

produces localized pain) and trigger points (sustained manual pressure resulting in pain referred to another area).

The aetiology of tension-type headache is likely to be multifactorial. There is a genetic predisposition, but environmental factors are also important. In addition to anxiety and depression, stressful life circumstances may play a part. The pathophysiology is unclear. The theory of increased scalp muscle tension has not been substantiated (Anderson and Frank, 1981).

Chronic tension-type headache usually evolves from the episodic form. It is speculated that prolonged painful input from the periphery causes central sensitization. A self-perpetuating disturbance is then established, with all peripheral afferents, including normal proprioception, being capable of causing pain.

Chronic head pain may also attend excessive and prolonged analgesic use (rebound headache). On cessation of such use, such patients may be completely headache-free, or headache may return episodically.

Diagnostic criteria for episodic tension-type headache (IHS, 1988)

A. At least ten previous headache episodes fulfilling the following criteria:
B. Headache lasting 30 min to 7 days
C. At least two of the following characteristics
   • pressing/tightening (non-pulsating quality)
   • mild to moderate severity
   • bilateral location
   • no aggravation by walking stairs or similar routine physical activity.
D. Both of the following:
   • No nausea or vomiting (anorexia may occur)
   • Photophobia and phonophobia are absent (one but not the other may be present).
E. History, physical examination and special investigations (as necessary) exclude other diagnoses.

Diagnostic criteria for chronic tension-type headache (IHS, 1988)

As for episodic tension-type headache, except that the headache occurs $\geq$ 15 days per month for 6 months.

Management

Overt depression and anxiety disorders must be diagnosed and treated appropriately.

The condition may be explained to the patient as a disturbance of the central pain-modulating system, such that normally innocuous stimuli are perceived as painful, with the secondary development of muscle tension, anxiety and depression. Advise that cure is rare but that control is usually attained.

Eliminate aggravating factors, especially analgesic abuse. Female sex hormones, particularly the combined pill, but also the progesterone-only pill, have been implicated, and discontinuation for a trial period of three months may be helpful. While 'stress' may play an aetiological role, it is impossible to live a totally stress-free life, and stress-reduction strategies rarely provide a complete answer. It is best to recommend adequate sleep and exercise.

Relaxation therapy, biofeedback and special exercise regimens have shown promise in some small trials. However, it is difficult to recommend such treatments, particularly at public expense, without convincing double-blind trials. Psychotherapy may help in the resolution of distressing issues.

Mertin (1993) provides an overview of the psychophysiological distinctions between the muscle tension and vascular headache and the treatment implications. Suggestions on psychological management are provided.

Mild analgesics (paracetamol 500–1000 mg) and NSAIDs (ibuprofen 400 mg) are recommended in acute episodic tension-type headache. Opioids are to be avoided. Anxiolytics are also better avoided, unless there are clear indications of anxiety. Patients must be made aware of the possible consequences of chronic medication use.

Tricyclics are the drug of choice in the prophylaxis. Amitriptyline 75 to 150 mg per day is recommended. The specific serotonin reuptake inhibitors (SSRIs) have not been shown to have the same effect.

Cluster headache

Cluster headache is categorized by a constant unilateral orbital localization, and predominantly occurs in young men. The pain is felt deep in and around the eye. It is intense and not usually throbbing. There may be radiation to the cheek, ear or other parts of the head.

The headache tends to commence about an hour after the onset of sleep. It usually recurs nightly (often at exactly the same time) for periods of six weeks or more. Periods of freedom may be of months or years; however, a small proportion may not remit.

The pain and associated features, which may include conjunctival injection, lacrimation, blocked nostril and others listed as diagnostic criteria, last about 45 minutes. The same-side temporal artery may become prominent and tender during an attack. The skin of the face and scalp may also be hyperalgesic.

The presentation of cluster headache is sufficiently typical that it permits a clinical diagnosis without additional investigations.

Prodromal symptoms may be present. They start minutes before the pain, and include sensations in the head and neck, alimentary symptoms and mood alterations.

Alcohol is known to precipitate attacks during active periods, but not during remissions.

The cause and mechanism of cluster

headache are unknown (Adams et al, 1997). Theories have included (1) paroxysmal parasympathetic discharge mediated through the greater superficial petrosal nerve and sphenopalatine ganglion; (2) swelling of the internal carotid artery in the canal through which it ascends in the petrous portion of the temporal bone; (3) dysregulation of hypothalamic mechanisms governing circadian rhythm; and (4) spontaneous release of histamine.

Diagnostic criteria for cluster headache (IHS, 1988)

A. At least five attacks satisfying the following criteria:
B. Severe unilateral orbital, supraorbital, or temporal pain lasting 15 to 80 minutes without treatment.
C. Headache is associated with at least one of the following signs, which have to be present on the pain side:
   - Conjunctival injection
   - Lacrimation
   - Nasal congestion
   - Rhinorrhoea
   - Forehead and facial swelling
   - Miosis
   - Ptosis
   - Eyelid oedema.
D. Frequency of attacks: from one every other day to eight per day.
E. Not due to another disorder.

Management

The patient should be advised that the condition is not associated with structural disease, and reassured that treatment is available to abort and prevent attacks.

Alcohol should be avoided during cluster periods. Afternoon naps should be avoided because they precipitate attacks.

Acute treatment

1. *Oxygen*
Oxygen inhalation aborts acute attacks. 100% oxygen is administered at 7 L per minute. Over 90% of individuals are reported to have relief in less than 10 minutes, and 100% have relief within 15 minutes. There are no side-effects, and oxygen is not contraindicated in any condition (unlike ergotamine). Tanks and regulators can be rented from suppliers.

2. *Sumatriptan*
Sumatriptan 6 mg by subcutaneous injection has been found effective and free of serious side-effects. Generally, no more than two injections in 24 hours. Sumatriptan has been found to be more convenient than oxygen by some patients. Sumatriptan 100 mg orally may also be effective.

3. *Naproxen*
Naproxen 500 mg may be useful as first aid in acute attacks, before other arrangements are made. Naproxen 500 mg twice daily may reduce attacks during the expected period.

Prophylaxis

1. *Lithium carbonate*

Lithium carbonate is recommended (Kudrow, 1980). The average dose is 1 g per day, which can be given in a single dose at night. However, dosage is determined by serum level, the range being 0.8–1.2 mM. Serum steady state is not reached for 5 days, blood to be taken 12 hours after last ingestion. Baseline thyroid function tests and urea and electrolyte levels are necessary. When used with a diuretic there may be retention of lithium and depletion of sodium, necessitating the close monitoring of electrolytes. Reversible hypothyroidism may develop, and can be treated by withdrawal of lithium or addition of thyroid hormone. There may be polyuria and polydipsia. Lithium should be avoided during the first trimester of pregnancy. While there may be some annoying side-effects, lithium is generally free of major adverse effects.

2. *Verapamil*

Verapamil commenced at a low dose and titrated to 320 mg per day in divided doses is recommended. Although the physiological effect is rapid, the maximal clinical effect may be delayed for some weeks.

3. *Naproxen*

Naproxen 500 mg twice daily may be effective. It is relatively straightforward to use, but the evidence for efficacy in prophylaxis is not well established.

Headache from cervical pathology

Headache from cervical pathology is rare. While being listed in newspaper advertisements posted by spinal manipulation exponents, it receives little space in certain classic works on pain (Bonica, 1990) and neurology (Adams et al, 1997).

Gobel and Edmeads (2000) list the cervical conditions that are accepted as the cause of headache: developmental abnormalities, tumours, Paget's disease, rheumatoid arthritis and craniocervical dystonia. These will be suggested by the history and stigmata of the underlying diseases. There is controversy as to whether disc disease and spondylosis, or 'whiplash' injury, cause headache.

Diagnostic criteria for headache associated with disorders of the cervical spine (IHS, 1988)

A. Pain is localized to the neck and occipital region. May project to forehead, orbital region, temples, vertex, or ears.

B. Pain is precipitated or aggravated by special neck movements or sustained neck pressure.

C. At least one of the following occurs:
- Resistance to or limitation of passive neck movements
- Changes in neck muscle contour,

texture, tone, or response to active and passive stretching and contraction.

- Abnormal tenderness of neck muscles.

D. Radiological examination reveals at least one of :

- Movement abnormalities in flexion and extension
- Abnormal posture
- Fractures, congenital abnormalities, tumours, RA, or other distinct pathology (not spondylosis or osteochondrosis).

Management

Causes should be identified and treated. Symptomatic pharmacological, surgical and chiropractic treatments do not produce lasting relief. Physiotherapy, muscle relaxation and psychotherapy may provide temporary relief.

It has been claimed that ipsilateral blockades of the C2 root of the occipital nerve may allow differentiation between headache due to irritation of the C2 nerve root and primary headache, such as migraine and tension-type headache. However, the effect is short-lived and the differentiation can be achieved on history (Gobel and Edmeads, 2000).

Craniocervical dystonia is a disorder that calls for special skills and experience, including the use of intramuscular injection of botulinum, thalamotomy and nerve resection.

Symptomatic treatment may be achieved

with paracetamol, NSAIDs or tramadol (up to 400 mg/day). Tramadol may cause gastrointestinal side-effects and sweating, and should be used with caution in combination with serotonin-enhancing antidepressants, because of the potential for the serotonin syndrome (characterized by restlessness, myoclonus, diaphoresis, tremor and mental status changes, such as confusion). Continuous use of analgesics should be avoided, owing to the danger of worsening the headache. Opioid substances are best avoided. A trial of TCAs (amitriptyline 25–50 mg/day) is worthy of consideration (adverse effects are mentioned above).

References

Adams R, Victor M, Ropper A. *Principles of Neurology*, 6th edn. McGraw-Hill, New York, 1997.

Anderson C, Frank R. Migraine and tension headache: Is there a physiological difference? *Headache* 1981; 21: 63–GGG.

Bonica J. *The Management of Pain*, 2nd edn. Lea & Febiger, Philadelphia, 1990.

Gobel H, Edmeads J. Disorders of the skull and cervical spine. In: Olesen J, Tfelt-Hansen P, Welch K (eds) *The Headaches*. Lippincott Williams and Wilkins, Philadelphia, 2000; 891–8.

Hassan H, Bastani B, Gellens M. Successful treatment of normeperidine neurotoxicity by hemodialysis. *American Journal of Kidney Disease* 2000; 35: 146–9.

IHS (Headache Classification Committee of the

International Headache Society). Classification and diagnostic criteria for headache disorders, cranial neuralgias and facial pain. *Cephalgia* 1988; 8(Suppl 7): 1–96.

Iversen H, Nielsen T, Olesen J. Arterial responses during migraine headache. *Lancet* 1990; 336: 837–FFF

Kudrow L. *Cluster Headache: Mechanisms and Management.* Oxford University Press, Oxford, 1980.

Lance J. *The Mechanisms and Management of Headache,* 5th edn. Butterworth-Heinemann, Boston, 1993.

Leao A. Spreading depression of activity in cerebral cortex. *Journal of Neurophysiology* 1944; 7: 359–KKK

Mertin P. *Psychological Management of Chronic Headaches.* Guilford, New York, 1993.

Olesen J, Tfelt-Hansen P, Welch K. *The Headaches,* 2nd edn. Lippincott Williams and Wilkins, Philadelphia, 2000.

Rasmussen B. Migraine and tension-type headache in a general population: precipitating factors, female hormones, sleep pattern and relation to lifestyle. *Pain* 1993; 53: 65–72.

Rasmussen B, Jensen R, Schroll M, Olsen J. Epidemiology of headache in a general population – a prevalence study. *Journal of Epidemiology* 1991; 44: 1147–57.

Taylor H. *The Nuprin Pain Report.* Lewis Harris and Associates, New York, 1985.

Wadsworth M, Butterfield W, Blaney R. Health and sickness. The choice of treatment. In *Perception of Illness and Use of Services in an Urban Community.* Tavistock, London, 1971.

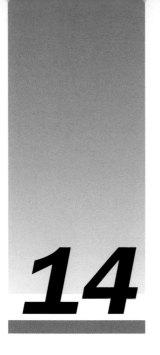

Low back pain and sciatica

'The trouble with being a hypochondriac these days is that antibiotics have cured all the good diseases.'

Caskie Stinnett

This book deals predominantly with chronic pain. When considering back pain, however, the acute condition is also discussed, as optimal treatment in the early stages may help prevent the chronic condition. 'Acute' is generally applied to a duration of less than 4 weeks, 'subacute', to 4 to 12 weeks, and 'chronic' is to durations of greater than 12 weeks.

'Back pain' refers to symptoms in the spinal and paraspinal region. It has an annual prevalence of 15–20% and is the second most common symptom leading to medical consultation (respiratory symptoms occupying first place). 'Sciatica' is pain radiating down the posterior or lateral aspect of the leg, often to the ankle or foot. It is usually due to nerve-root involvement. One per cent of patients with acute back pain have nerve-root symptoms. Back pain and sciatica are expensive to the individual and the community, and are the cause of great suffering and disability.

The important issues in back pain and sciatica include the facts that (1) the vast majority of cases are the result of benign non-specific mechanical problems; (2) acute non-specific mechanical pain improves in one month in 75–90% of cases, and sciatica improves in six weeks in more than 50% of cases; (3) very rarely are these pains the result of serious progressive disorders; (4) a short list of symptoms is available, 'red flags', that warn of serious progressive conditions; (5) a comprehensive history and physical examination, with particular attention to 'red flags', is the starting-point; (6) when there is clear evidence of a serious, progressive disorder, immediate special investigation and referral are appropriate; (7) when there is suspicion of a serious progressive condition, regular, close review by the primary care physician is appropriate and will clarify the situation; (8) the primary care physician is well placed to manage the majority of cases of back pain with and without sciatica; (9) the important features of acute management are rapid return to normal activities, education of the patient about the condition and mild analgesia as required; (10) special investigations should be used sparingly, and only when there is a clear indication; (11) chronic back pain has a poor prognosis and is often associated with psychosocial and compensation issues; and (12) rapid resumption of daily activities, the avoidance of powerful analgesics and modification of the workplace may help prevent the chronic condition.

The differential diagnosis

The differential diagnosis of low back pain has been divided into mechanical and non-mechanical conditions (Deyo, 1986). The mechanical conditions include muscle and ligament strains, degenerative disease of the spine, facet joint disease, bulging and herniated disc, fracture, spondylolisthesis and spinal stenosis (narrowing of the spinal canal).

It is difficult to distinguish between the mechanical problems by physical examination and diagnostic testing. Imaging is frequently unhelpful; when imaging reveals pathology, it is often impossible to be certain that a candidate finding is causing a particular pain (Jensen et al, 1994). For example, 60% of pain free imaged individuals over the age of 60 years demonstrate disc degeneration (Wiesel et al, 1984; Powell et al, 1986).

As was mentioned in the earlier chapter on Plasticity and neuropathic pain, nociceptive input has been associated with plastic changes in the spinal cord and brain such that the nervous system may become sensitized and respond to mild nociceptive and non-nociceptive input as though it were strongly nociceptive. Using magnetic resonance spectroscopy, Grachev et al (2000) demonstrated reductions in N-acetyl aspartate and glucose in the dorsolateral prefrontal cortex of patients with back pain. These changes in the brain chemistry substantiate the view that back pain is associated with brain changes, and raise the possibility that sensitization may occur.

The presence or absence of neurological symptoms is a straightforward and useful distinction. Sciatica may compound back pain and is usually associated with disc herniation, but may also accompany other pathology, including spinal stenosis and degenerative bony conditions (Atlas and Deyo, 2001).

The non-mechanical conditions can be divided into those that directly involve the spine, such as neoplasia, infection and inflammatory arthritis, and those that involve other systems, such as vascular disease and diseases of pelvic, renal and gastrointestinal organs. These are all uncommon (Deyo et al, 1992).

Clinical course of benign back pain and sciatica

The clinical course of the serious progressive conditions will depend on the nature of the specific condition. Mechanical problems are by far the most common causes of back pain, and the majority are non-specific and self-limiting (Atlas and Deyo, 2001). Seventy-five to 90% of such cases improve in one month (Croft et al, 1998) and more than 50% of sciatica cases improve in six weeks (Andersson et al, 1983).

The above figures are encouraging, and support the conservative approach. Nevertheless, at least 5% of those with back

pain still have symptoms at three months (Frymoyer et al, 1983), at least 10% report persistent symptoms at one year, and 25–50% report relapse within one year (Croft et al, 1998). This relatively small group of patients with chronic pain accounts for the greater part of disability, compensation and public costs in general.

The diagnostic process

The assessment of back pain is daunting, as the differential diagnosis is extensive and includes serious progressive conditions. Guidelines have been developed that protect both the patient and the doctor (Bigos et al, 1994). The first task is to identify the serious progressive conditions and investigate and refer as appropriate. A thorough history and physical examination, taking account of a short list of symptoms, 'red flags', will achieve this end with reasonable sensitivity and certainty (Deyo et al, 1992).

Red flags

1. Recent severe trauma
2. Weight loss, night sweats, fever
3. Past history of carcinoma, steroids, IV drug use
4. Severe night pain
5. Structural deformity
6. Progressive neurological deficits
7. Inflammatory character pain
8. Features of cauda equina syndrome

(urinary retention, saddle anaesthesia, bilateral neurological symptoms and signs)

Not considered a red flag, but worth remembering is the fact that complaints of back pain in the presence of normal movements and the absence of tenderness suggest a visceral or vascular source of pain. In practice, most of the red flags noted by clinicians prove to be false positives; but caution is recommended.

The physical examination should commence with the patient standing and unclothed. The important features are posture, flexibility and tenderness. Straight-leg raising in lying is a good screening test for nerve-root complications. A history of sciatica or straight-leg raising limited by pain to less than 60 degrees calls for a more detailed neurological examination of the lower limb. Full details are available in texts on physical examination and neurology. In 98% of cases, disc herniation involves the L5 and S1 nerves (Spangfort, 1972). Screening for L5 pathology includes extension of the great toe and walking on the heels, and loss of sensation on the dorsum of the foot. Screening for S1 pathology includes walking on the toes, decreased sensation on the lateral aspect of the sole, and reduced ankle reflex.

When there is strong evidence of a serious progressive condition, immediate referral to a specialist is appropriate. Whether special investigations are conducted will depend on a range of circumstances, but this can usually be discussed with, and performed on the way to, the specialist. When a red flag condition is suspected, it is reasonable to schedule further visits and keep the case under close review (Bogduk, 1999).

Special investigations

It is important to order special investigations only when the results will influence treatment. Imaging studies may not be helpful, as findings are poorly associated with symptoms. The most common causes of nerve root irritation, herniated disc and spinal stenosis cannot be demonstrated with plain radiographs.

CT and MRI studies should be ordered when the history and examination strongly suggest a serious progressive disorder such as cauda equina syndrome, infection or tumour. When sciatica is probably due to a herniated disc or spinal stenosis, and neurological signs are slight, early imaging is unnecessary, as patients can be expected to recover with conservative management (Atlas and Deyo, 2001). If improvement is slow with conservative treatment, imaging studies should be conducted. However, in chronic back pain, extensive evaluations usually show no surgically correctable lesions (Frymoyer, 1988).

The patient may have expectations that imaging will be performed. When appropriate, it will be possible to reassure the patient, and not ordering special investigations may reassure that this is a benign condition, familiar to the doctor. Alternatively, it may not be possible to retain the confidence of the patient without performing some screening tests. It is not uncommon to encounter patents who have had repeated imaging studies only months or even weeks apart, sometimes ordered by the same doctor. Unless there are excellent indications that change has occurred, repeat studies cannot be justified.

Routine laboratory tests are not needed. When other than benign mechanical conditions are considered, erythrocyte sedimentation rate (ESR), full blood count and urinalysis are useful and relatively inexpensive screening tests. Testing for the HLA-B27 antigen has been useful in suspected ankylosing spondylitis.

Nuclear medicine and clinical neurophysiology studies are better conducted in collaboration with a specialist.

Management in the acute stage

The conservative approach emphasizes the need for reassurance, and education of the patient regarding the nature of the condition and its probable prognosis, and the opportunity for recovery. Extended bed rest is unhelpful. In both back pain (Malmivaara et al, 1995) and sciatica (Vroomen et al, 1999), return to usual activities has produced better outcomes than formal bed rest. It is recommended that bed rest should be available as necessary and that activities that promote pain should be avoided.

In the acute situation, the patient is in pain and movement makes it worse. This is a most distressing situation. The patient fears the pain and fears that it will not be relieved and may even get worse, and further, that an inability to perform the usual duties will have dire financial and social consequences for the individual and the family. Fear of pain and movement is a major cause of chronicity (Croft et al, 1995), and has been discussed at length in an earlier chapter. Thus the importance of early reassurance, an explanation of the nature of the condition and an exposition of the rationale of treatment cannot be overemphasized.

Psychosocial factors frequently play a role in the persistence of back pain and disability. Accordingly, experts recommend identifying, early in the acute stage, those patients with psychosocial risk factors, in the hope that appropriate management will prevent the chronic condition. While this approach makes sense and guides modern management, the study has not yet been performed that substantiates the approach. It is relevant, however, that studies of rapid return to usual activities have had favourable outcomes. This process protects income, status and self-esteem. It also helps to avoid conflict between patient, employer and insurer, and resentment, anger and protracted legal battles. Further, early return to work is associated with less use of problematic medication, and consequently, less risk of drug-use complications.

Other risk factors for persistent symptoms include a history of painful disorders, depression, personality disorder, substance abuse and current litigation and dissatisfaction with work (Andersson et al, 1983; Deyo and Diehl, 1988). Psychiatric, social work and occupational therapy assessments should be conducted as appropriate. Psychiatric disorder, such as depression, should be vigorously treated. For the patient who finds work unrewarding, it may be possible for the employer to provide alternative, more satisfying duties. The occupational therapist may choose to take part in such negotiations.

Medication in the acute stage should be limited, whenever possible, to non-steroidal anti-inflammatory drugs (NSAIDs), mild analgesics such as paracetamol, and tricyclic antidepressants. When stronger analgesics are necessary, non-addictive tramadol may have a place. Avoidance of potent opioids and benzodiazepines, whenever possible, will help to prevent addiction and iatrogenic complications.

Referral for specialist consultation is appropriate when there is good evidence of serious progressive disorder or recovery is unacceptably slow and psychosocial factors can be excluded as influential factors. While going to surgery too soon should be avoided, delaying herniated disc surgery beyond 12 weeks has been found to compromise outcome (Weber, 1978). However, no more than 5 to 10 per cent of patients with unremitting sciatica require operation (Frymoyer, 1988). One study found that surgical treatment of lumbar disc herniation produced a better functional ability and fewer symptoms than non-surgical management at one and two years, but that this was no longer evident at four and ten years (Weber, 1978).

Physical treatments such as spinal manipulation, facet joint injection, epidural steroid injection and ligamentous injection and acupuncture are said to be of value, but others claim efficacy has yet to be proved (Atlas and Deyo, 2001).

Management of the chronic stage

Typically, patients with chronic back pain have suffered a benign mechanical problem. Some have received back surgery but have continued to suffer pain and disability. It is important to treat existing mechanical problems, but it is unwise to pursue a physical lesion relentlessly.

As emphasized above, it is important to try to identify those cases at risk of developing chronic problems and to take preventive action. This is the theoretical ideal, which can be difficult to achieve in practice. Psychiatric consultation is indicated, and existing psychiatric disorders should be treated.

In the chronic stage, efforts to reassure and educate the patient regarding the role of fear of pain and movement in perpetuating the condition should be redoubled. Patients often believe that pain is an indication that their body is undergoing further damage, and this discourages them from any activity. Consequently, they lose muscle strength, joint flexibility and aerobic fitness, which further increases the likelihood of experiencing pain. Patients need to learn that while acute pain indicates damage and serves to immobilize the injured part, chronic pain does not indicate new damage – it serves no useful purpose, and is, in fact, maladaptive, as it discourages return to normal function. Patients are encouraged gradually to increase their daily activity. However, they are also taught to pace themselves, meaning that they are taught to avoid exerting themselves to the degree that will cause a flare-up of symptoms. Thus, 'pacing' means dividing tasks into manageable quantities that extend the patient, perhaps on subsequent days, without causing setbacks. Psychological techniques including relaxation and cognitive restructuring may have a place in reducing anxiety and chronic pain. Multidisciplinary programmes offer advantages (Nicholas et al, 2000). Massage may be superior to acupuncture and self-care

education in the short term, and may be superior to acupuncture at one-year follow-up (Cherkin et al, 2001).

Chronic pain may be helped by medication. The patient needs to understand and accept that medication can usually provide moderate symptomatic relief, but that complete eradication of pain is unlikely. Side-effects frequently cause problems; some information on reducing side-effects can be found in the final chapter on Pharmacotherapy. It is better, when possible, to avoid opioid use because of the problems of tolerance and addiction.

Symptoms accompanying chronic pain include fear (anxiety), depression, insomnia and irritability. It is often very difficult, in particular cases, to disentangle and make definitive statements about these symptoms. The most parsimonious approach is to regard them as components of a depressive syndrome, such as major depressive disorder, which might be expected to develop secondary to unrelenting pain. However, clinical experience is that some of these symptoms can present alone, or in combination, without being part of a depressive syndrome. This issue has not been fully researched, but clearly, insomnia and irritability may present alone or in combination, in the absence of a full depressive syndrome. Again, it is reasonable to expect these symptoms as a consequence of unrelenting pain. In practice, patients often complain most about their irritability. This is because of angry outbursts toward family members, who have been loving and supportive, which leave the patient feeling regretful and self-critical.

The above paragraph is, to some extent, an academic exercise, as the antidepressants are useful and recommended for the management of anxiety, depression, insomnia and irritability, whether as separate symptoms or as part of a depressive syndrome. When the full depressive syndrome is present, the normal antidepressant dose is usually required. However, symptomatic relief from anxiety, insomnia and irritability is usually achieved at smaller doses. The choice of antidepressant is important. While the newer antidepressants, venlafaxine and the selective serotonin reuptake inhibitors (SSRIs) such as fluoxetine, may be useful in full doses in the treatment of the depressive syndrome, they are less useful in the symptomatic treatment of anxiety, insomnia and irritability. In symptomatic treatment, the older, tricyclic antidepressants (TCAs), are more useful. The TCAs cause dry mouth and other anticholinergic side-effects; but this may be minimized by using smaller doses of the more tolerable agents, such as nortriptyline. Twenty-five or 50 mg of amitriptyline or nortriptyline will greatly assist pain-related insomnia, and 10 or 25 mg once or twice per day will assist anxiety and irritability.

The TCAs also have an important, first-line role in the analgesia of back pain

(Fishbain, 2000). Thus, the TCAs may have multiple benefits in the management of this condition.

The anticonvulsants have traditionally been recommended in the treatment of neuropathic pain. However, in practice they are also used in the management of chronic back pain, irrespective of the possibility of a neuropathic contribution. In view of the wide range of actions of these drugs, Caraceni et al (2000) speculate that the anticonvulsants may prove to have a wide range of applications in pain. In chronic back pain, as with the TCAs, the anticonvulsants have the advantage of beneficial effects in anxiety and depression. Carbamazepine and sodium valproate are well established in the treatment of chronic pain; however, gabapentin is now being used, and appears to be as effective, but with less troublesome side-effects.

The NSAIDs have a place in chronic back pain, particularly where degenerative conditions contribute. They have troublesome gastrointestinal effects, but the cyclooxygenase-2 inhibitors, such as celecoxib, have relatively fewer.

When opioids are being contemplated, tramadol deserves consideration. It displays both weak opioid and monaminergic actions. It is thought to be free of euphoria, withdrawal and addiction problems. There is minimal respiratory depression, but nausea and somnolence are common side-effects. In at least one study benefit has been demonstrated in chronic low back pain (Schnitzer et al, 2000).

The use of opioids for non-cancer pain remains controversial, but there is good evidence that they relieve chronic back pain (Jamison et al, 1998). In comparisons of populations who receive and do not receive opioids, it emerges that the factor that determines the decision to provide opioids is not the quantity of pain suffered, but the amount of emotional distress experienced. It is important, therefore, specifically to assess the mental state and reduce emotional distress with antidepressants and psychological therapies before resorting to the opioids. Once the decision is made, the choice of agent will depend on experience and availability. An acceptable approach is the combination of a long-acting medication taken regularly (daily or twice daily) and a short-acting medication taken as required, for breakthrough pain. See the final chapter on pharmacotherapy for details.

When oral opioids are deemed to have failed, in highly specialized centres devices such as morphine pumps and epidural stimulators may be implanted. There are no controlled trials that support the use of these devices.

References

Andersson G, Svensson H-O, Oden A. The intensity of work recovery in low back pain. *Spine* 1983; 8: 880–4.

Atlas S, Deyo R. Evaluating and managing acute low back pain in the primary care setting. *Journal of General Internal Medicine* 2001; 16: 120–31.

Bigos S, Bowyer O, Braen G. Acute low back problems in adults. *Clinical Practice Guidelines no. 14.* Rockville, MD, Department of Health and Human Services, 1994. (AHCPR publication no. 95–0642.)

Bogduk N. Management of low back pain. In: *Update in the Management of Musculoskeletal Pain.* Alpha Biomedical Communications, Darlinghurst, 1999; 85–102.

Caraceni, A, Cheville A, Portenoy R. Pain management: pharmacological and nonpharmacological treatments. In: Massie MJ (ed) *Pain: What Psychiatrists Need to Know.* (Review of Psychiatry Series, Vol. 19, No 2; Oldham J and Riba M, series eds). American Psychiatric Press, Washington, DC, 2000; 23–88.

Cherkin D, Eisenberg D, Sherman K, Barlow W, Kaptchuk T, Street J, Deyo R. Randomized trial comparing traditional Chinese medical acupuncture, therapeutic massage, and self-care education for chronic low back pain. *Archives of Internal Medicine* 2001; 161: 1081–8.

Croft P, Papageorgiou A, Ferry S, Thomas E, Jayson M, Silman A. Psychological distress and low back pain: evidence from a prospective study in the general population. *Spine* 1995; 20: 2731–7.

Croft P, Macfarlane G, Papageorgiou A, Thomas E, Silman A. Outcome of low back pain in general practice: a prospective study. *British Medical Journal* 1998; 316: 1356–9.

Deyo R. Early diagnostic evaluation of low back pain. *Journal of General Internal Medicine* 1986; 1: 328–38.

Deyo R, Diehl A. Psychosocial predictors of

disability in patients with low back pain. *Journal of Rheumatology* 1988; 15: 1557–64.

Deyo R, Rainville J, Kent D. What can the history and physical examination tell us about low back pain? *Journal of the American Medical Association* 1992; 268: 760–4.

Fishbain D. Evidence-based data on pain relief with antidepressants. *Annals of Medicine* 2000; 32: 305–16.

Frymoyer J, Pope M, Clements J, Wilder D, MacPherson B, Ashikaga T. Risk factors in low-back pain: an epidemiological survey. *Journal of Bone and Joint Surgery* [Am] 1983; 64-A: 213–18.

Frymoyer J. Back pain and sciatica. *New England Journal of Medicine* 1988; 318: 291–300.

Grachev I, Fredrickson B, Apkarian A. Abnormal brain chemistry in chronic back pain: an in vivo proton magnetic resonance spectroscopy study. *Pain* 2000; 89: 7–18.

Jamison R, Raymond S, Slawsby E, Nedeljkovic S, Katz N. Opioid therapy for chronic noncancer back pain. A randomized prospective study. *Spine* 1998; 23: 2591–600.

Jensen M, Brant-Zawadzki M, Obuchowski N, Modic M, Malkasian D, Ross J. Magnetic resonance imaging of the lumbar spine in people without back pain. *New England Journal of Medicine* 1994; 331: 69–73.

Malmivaara A, Hakkinen U, Aro T. The treatment of acute low back pain – bed rest, or ordinary activity. *New England Journal of Medicine* 1995; 332: 351–5.

Nicholas M, Molloy A, Tonkin L, Beeston L. *Manage Your Pain: Practical and Positive Ways of Adapting to Chronic Pain.* Australian Broadcasting Commission, Sydney, 2000.

Powell M, Wilson M, Szypryt P, Symonds E, Worthington B. Prevalence of lumbar disc degeneration observed by magnetic resonance in symptomless women. *Lancet* 1986; 2: 1366–7.

Schnitzer T, Gray W, Paster R, Kamin M. Efficacy of tramadol in treatment of chronic low back pain. *Journal of Rheumatology* 2000; 27: 772–8.

Spangfort E. The lumbar disk herniation: a computer-aided analysis of 2,504 operations. *Acta Orthopaedica Scandinavica* [Suppl] 1972; 142: 1–95.

Vroomen P, de Krom M, Wilmink J, Kester A, Knottnerus J. Lack of effectiveness of bed rest for sciatica. *New England Journal of Medicine* 1999; 340: 418–23.

Weber H. Lumbar disc herniation: a prospective study of prognostic factors including a *controlled trial.* Part I. *Journal of Oslo City Hospital* 1978; 28: 33–61.

Wiesel S, Tsourmas N, Feffer H, Citrin C, Patronas N. A study of computer-assisted topography. I. The incidence of positive CAT scans in an asymptomatic group of patients. *Spine* 1984; 9: 549–51.

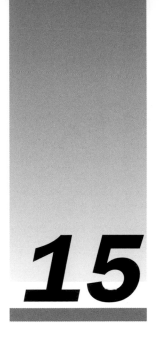

Pharmacotherapy

'The desire to take medicine is perhaps the greatest feature which distinguishes man from the animals.'

Sir William Osler 1904

Pain relief may be sought from a range of non-pharmacological procedures (relaxation therapy, hypnosis, CBT, acupuncture, and invasive techniques), but pharmacotherapy remains the most widely used and effective component, and is usually indispensable to chronic pain management.

Patients may be reluctant to take medication. There are pragmatic concerns regarding adverse effects and addiction and cultural concerns. Many cultures view the origin of pain in religious terms or maintain attitudes that idolize pain. They equate the acceptance of pain with faith and the toleration of pain with character strength. It is the task of the clinician to help the patient avoid adverse effects, drug abuse and unnecessary suffering.

Adverse effects in general

Adverse effects are frequent and may lead to non-compliance and subsequent treatment failure. The clinician should be aware of the potential adverse effects of each medication and monitor patient progress. One current view, supported by the patients' rights movements and legal systems, is that the patient must be informed about every known adverse effect of every medication. Another view is that patients are ill prepared to weigh the risks and benefits of specific medications. Exhaustive information may increase patient apprehension and the rate of detection/reporting of adverse effects, for no clinical gain. Thus some recommend giving only a brief account of possible adverse effects, encouraging contact at the first sign of problems, and arranging a follow-up visit for the near future. At follow-up, the clinician asks non-leading questions about the body systems that may be affected. It is legally safer for the clinician to take the comprehensive warning approach, which is often less beneficial for the patient.

It is sometimes possible to reduce the impact of adverse effects. Always use the minimal effective dose. Commencing at full dose produces the strongest adverse effects. This frightens and discourages and carries the strongest likelihood of rejection of both this medication in particular and all other medications. As a general rule, start with low doses and gradually increase. This allows the patients gradually to become aware of and gradually to accept adverse effects, and for physiological adjustments that will minimize them. Some adverse effects occur much less

frequently with gradual introduction. For example, carbamazepine and lamotrigene are much less likely to cause characteristic skin reactions if they are introduced slowly.

When a patient is troubled by a particular adverse effect, it may be possible to change to another medication in the same family that is less troublesome. For example, when a first-generation tricyclic antidepressant (TCA; e.g. amitriptyline) produces an unacceptably dry mouth, a second-generation TCA (e.g. desipramine), which has less anticholinergic action, may be an answer.

Adverse effects may also be diminished by altering the time of administration. When possible, give the majority of the sedating drugs of the regimen at night. This depends on the purpose and half-life of the medication. Amitriptyline (half life 21 hours) given for depression, can be given all at night, while codeine (half life 2.9 hours) given for pain, is better given throughout the day. Likewise, activating agents such as stimulants should be given in the morning. Different patients may report different sedating or alerting effects from the same medication. A careful history will reveal the problem and the necessary accommodation can be made.

The use of multiple pharmacological agents for the same or concurrent illnesses increases the likelihood of adverse effects. Clinicians need to be informed regarding interactions that cause adverse effects or reduce the efficacy of specific agents. For example, selective serotonin reuptake inhibitors (SSRIs) will raise the blood level of concomitantly administered TCAs, and carbamazepine will lower the blood level of a range of drugs, including oral contraceptives.

Pharmacological agents introduced to correct adverse effects initiated by therapeutic agents may introduce their own adverse effects. For example, choline esters introduced to correct the effects of anticholinergic drugs may themselves cause tremor, diarrhoea, abdominal cramps, and excessive eye watering; misoprostol, a prostaglandin analogue used to prevent gastric ulceration by NSAIDs, may cause abdominal pain and diarrhoea. Inquiries regarding the concomitant use of over-the-counter medications, herbal remedies, caffeine, nicotine, and alcohol are mandatory.

In general, the elderly are at greater risk of adverse effects, and for them smaller medication doses are indicated.

Common adverse effects

1. Nausea and vomiting

Nausea and vomiting are common adverse effects of the opioids and the antiarrhythmics (mexiletine). The vomiting centre, which is situated in the brain stem, is stimulated by input from the chemoreceptor trigger zone, the vestibular system and the gastrointestinal tract. The chemoreceptor trigger zone is stimulated by the opioids. This stimulation is blocked by the antidopaminergics (metoclopramide and prochlorperazine) and the antiserotonergics (ondansetron). The vestibular system is stimulated by movement; thus it is better to rest than move during these periods. The sensitivity of the vestibular system can be reduced by anticholinergics (scopolamine and benztropine) and antihistamines (diphenhydramine). The opioids decrease the activity of the gastrointestinal tract, which produces abnormal feedback to the vomiting centre.

Metoclopramide 10 mg (up to 3 times daily, if necessary) is the treatment of choice, as it has a dopamine-blocking action and also increases gastrointestinal activity. Adverse effects include dystonic reactions (which may need treatment with an anticholinergic and/or benzodiazepine) and sedation.

Prochlorperazine 10 mg (up to 3 times daily) is a strong alternative. This may also cause dystonia and sedation. Ondansetron is a useful but expensive alternative that may cause headache and constipation. Diphenhydramine 25 mg (up to 4 times daily) is inexpensive, but will increase sedation.

Scopolamine patches have been recommended, but these are no longer available in some countries (including Australia).

2. Constipation

Constipation is a frequent consequence of anticholinergic activity, and of stimulation of mu and delta opioid receptors.

Helpful agents include the following:

Eat more fruit and drink larger amounts of water.
Fibre supplements (ispaghula, Fybogel; methylcellulose, Cellulone)
Faecal softener by mouth (docusate, Coloxyl). Faecal softeners stimulate intestinal secretions, which enter and soften the stool. Thus oral administration may not be effective for two or three days.
Peristaltic stimulant (sennosides a and b, Senokot)
Combinations of faecal softener and peristaltic stimulant are available.
Suppositories (glycerol; Glycerine Suppositories; docusate, Coloxyl Suppositories)
Enema (docusate; Coloxyl Enema)

Laxatives should be used with caution. They are contraindicated in suspected obstruction and certain other medical conditions. They may increase the absorption and hepatic uptake of other drugs. Continuous high-dose use may lead to dependence and should be avoided. However, regular intake of fibre supplement with faecal softener as required should be safe in the otherwise healthy individual.

Some tolerance develops to the effects of opioids on gastrointestinal motility; however, patients who take opioids chronically remain constipated.

Bethanechol has been suggested for anticholinergic constipation. This choline ester has been associated with adverse effects of asthma, hyperthyroidism, coronary insufficiency and peptic ulcer. Regular use for drug-induced constipation is not recommended; it is not particularly effective, and is therefore not worth the risk of further adverse effects.

Use of laxatives may be necessary where high-dose opioid use is unavoidable. In many cases it is possible to reduce or change the offending medication, and increased intake of fruit, water and some fibre supplement will be sufficient.

3. Pruritus

Pruritus results from spinal cord mu receptors. It is relieved by diphenhydramine 25 mg (up to 4 times daily).

4. Orthostatic hypotension

Orthostatic hypotension may result from blockade of alpha 1-adrenergic receptors. Affected patients should be advised to change posture slowly and to sit down immediately upon experiencing dizziness. Supportive stockings to prevent venous pooling are recommended by some authors, but are rarely used in clinical practice. Other measures may include adding salt to the diet, and the use of fludrocortisone. This adverse effect usually subsides over time.

Orthostatic hypotension may also result from opioid use. There is peripheral arteriolar and venous dilation, produced by several mechanisms, including provoked histamine release. There is also blunting of reflex vasoconstriction in response to plasma CO_2. There is no specific treatment; reduce the dose and consider an alternative analgesic agent.

5. Sedation

Sedation may result from stimulation of mu and kappa receptors by opioid drugs and stimulation of histamine receptors by antidepressant drugs.

Sedation due to opioid drugs in the terminally ill may be managed with a stimulant such as methylphenidate 5 mg (up to 3 times daily). For non-cancer chronic pain patients, however, the currently available stimulants, which are addictive and have other adverse effects, are not recommended. For these patients, dose reduction or changing to another opioid may be beneficial.

The tricyclic antidepressants (TCAs) are the most frequently used antidepressants for chronic pain patients, because they have an analgesic effect. This has not been satisfactorily demonstrated in the selective serotonin reuptake inhibitors (SSRIs). The SSRIs have insignificant sedative effects. If a TCA is being used for analgesic effects, and sedation is a problem, replacement with an SSRI cannot be recommended. Amitriptyline

is the most widely used TCA in pain management, but is the most sedating. Nortriptyline is a metabolite of amitriptyline. It is less sedating but retains analgesic effects, and can be used to replace the parent drug. Desipramine is a TCA that is stimulating in some individuals. It is not used extensively in pain management, where a degree of sedation is often valuable.

Where the antidepressant is being used exclusively in the treatment of depression, an SSRI will provide a non-sedating alternative.

6. Urinary retention

Urinary retention may result from the use of anticholinergic drugs. It is rare that active treatment is needed. Bethanechol has a good effect, and can be use in oral or in subcutaneous form in acute situations.

Urinary retention may occur when stimulation of the mu and delta opioid receptors inhibits the voiding reflex. Catheterization may be necessary in acute situations. Tolerance develops to the effect of opioids on the bladder.

7. Dry mouth

Dry mouth may be caused by anticholinergic drugs. Oral bethanechol has been suggested, but may cause other adverse effects. Some relief may be obtained from chewing sugarless gum or sweets. It is important to use sugarless products, as a dry mouth makes teeth particularly prone to caries. The cholinomimetic alkaloid pilocarpine used as a 1% solution mouthwash used three times daily has the advantage of being relatively effective; and, as a topical preparation, the risk of further adverse effects carried is slight. This use of pilocarpine is not listed in some authoritative pharmacological texts (Taylor, 1990).

8. Blurred vision

Blurred vision may be caused by anticholinergic drugs. Pilocarpine 1% one drop four times daily can be beneficial and is free of adverse effects. The frequency of application depends on the individual.

Miosis may result from stimulation of mu and kappa opioid receptors, but rarely impairs vision.

9. Sexual dysfunction

Sexual dysfunction (decreased libido, impotence, impaired ejaculation, inhibition of female orgasm) can be associated with a range of drugs acting on the nervous system.

Sexual dysfunction is an uncommon complication of analgesic use. Opioids inhibit the release of gonadotropin-releasing hormone (GnRH) and corticotropin-releasing factor (CRF) and increase the concentration of prolactin (PRL): thus sexual dysfunction is possible.

Sildenafil is effective in drug-induced impotence and impaired ejaculation and has relatively trivial adverse effects (most commonly, headache, flushing and dyspepsia). It may also have a place in the treatment of female sexual dysfunction. Bethanecol has been use for impotence. Neostigmine by mouth half an hour before sexual intercourse may help impaired ejaculation, but is no longer available in some countries (including Australia). Cyproheptadine as a regular morning dose, or one to two hours before anticipated sexual activity, may help inhibited orgasm (Grebb, 1995).

When sexual dysfunction is the adverse effect of an SSRI, the addition of a small dose of bupropion usually produces good results (Labbate and Pollack, 1994).

10. Gastric irritation and ulcer

Gastrointestinal (GI) symptoms occur in 10% of patients treated with traditional NSAIDs. Ulcers occur in 2%. GI symptoms are poor predictors, and haemorrhage and perforation of ulcers may occur without warning.

The analgesic properties of the NSAIDs result from inhibition of the enzyme cyclooxygenase (COX), which is central to the production of prostaglandins. COX exists in at least two physiological forms (COX-1 and COX-2). COX-1 inhibition is associated with GI (and renal) toxicity, while COX-2 inhibition reduces inflammation and pain.

Most currently used NSAIDs are non-specific inhibitors of both isoforms of COX. When using these, when symptoms or risk factors (past history, heavy alcohol use, older age) cause concern, gastroprotective therapy is indicated. Misoprostol (800 micrograms in divided doses), a prostaglandin analogue, reduces the incidence of ulcers. This treatment may lead to abdominal pain and diarrhoea. A proton pump inhibitor such as omeprazole (20 mg daily) or a histamine H_2 receptor antagonist such as cimetidine (400 mg in divided doses) may also be effective. Both are associated with a range of generally mild adverse effects.

With regard to gastric irritation and ulcer, the selective COX-2 inhibitors such as celecoxib have advantages. Where they can be afforded, such drugs are recommended.

11. Weight gain

Weight gain is a common and troublesome adverse effect of many drugs that act on the CNS. Fluid retention, increased appetite and caloric intake, dry mouth leading to frequent drinks, sedation and decreased exercise, and altered metabolism may all play a part.

The TCAs cause significant weight gain; the SSRIs cause little. When a TCA is being used for its analgesic effects, it cannot be replaced by an SSRI. However, when a TCA is being used exclusively as an antidepressant, and weight gain is a problem, replacement with an SSRI is recommended.

Among the antipsychotic drugs, olanzapine causes marked weight gain, while quetiapine causes almost none. The antihistamines are notorious for weight gain, and should be avoided as regular treatment where overweight is a problem.

Patients should attempt to restrict fats and carbohydrates. Where dry mouth is a problem, pilocarpine mouthwash may be useful, but most important is to alert the patient to the calorie content of drinks and encourage the drinking of plain water or other calorie-free beverages. The involvement of a dietician may be helpful. Exercise is encouraged. When weight gain has been unavoidable, discussions may help the patient accept this altered condition.

Opioids (opioid receptor actors)

The opioid drugs are the strongest analgesics available. They are similar to the endogenous opioids, the endorphins. The human has at least five opiate receptors (mu, kappa, sigma, delta, epsilon), which have different constellations of actions. The mu, kappa and delta receptors have analgesic effects. The mu receptor has euphoric and the kappa and sigma receptors have dysphoric effects. The mu, kappa and delta receptors cause respiratory depression, while the sigma receptor causes increased respiration.

Brain opiate receptors are mainly located

in the periaqueductal grey matter. Stimulation activates dorsal column noradrenaline and serotonin-transmitting neurones that inhibit afferent input in the dorsal horns. Spinal opiate receptors are mainly located in the dorsal horns. Their stimulation has a direct inhibitory effect on afferent transmission.

Tolerance, dependency and addiction

These conditions are poorly understood, a situation that creates difficulties for people with chronic pain and doctors alike. The principles are simple. They should be clearly communicated and understood, and returned to, should clinical practice become problematic.

Tolerance

Tolerance is the condition that a certain dose of medication produces a decreased effect following repeated administration. Consequently, a greater dose is thereafter required to achieve the desired effect. Tolerance is a normal, adaptive response to drugs, and is demonstrated in a wide range of animals. Various bodily changes may contribute to tolerance, including the induction of metabolizing enzymes, moderation via negative feedback of endocrine gland activity, and the alteration of receptor density in the 'plastic' nervous system.

Tolerance also develops to drugs other than the opioids. For example, carbamazepine doses have to be increased subsequent to the induction of metabolizing enzymes.

In humans tolerance to constipation does not develop. This means that the starting dose, or relatively small doses, continue to cause this problem. Fortunately, tolerance to respiratory depression and sedation develops over a few weeks, so that the starting dose, or another particular dose, will cease to cause these problems. However, at very high doses, tolerance finally ceases and the persistence of adverse effects prevents further dose escalation.

Tolerance to the euphoric effect develops in days to weeks. This is at the root of the psychological dependency of addiction, which will be discussed below. Where the euphoric effect is a primary goal, or becomes an important goal, tolerance will result in the seeking of higher doses.

Tolerance also, unfortunately, develops to the analgesic effects. However, clinically, this is usually a gradual process, and it is common for patients to remain on a stable dose for years (Brescia et al, 1992). There are a number of confounding factors. Rapid escalation of dose by the doctor encourages tolerance. On the other hand, requests from the patient for rapid escalation call for physical and mental re-evaluation. However, there is no ceiling effect, and as long as the adverse effects are tolerable, increasing the dose will restore the analgesic effect. When approaching very high doses, the clinician should involve colleagues in the decision to increase.

Tolerance is soon lost. This means that if opioids can be tapered and ceased for three or four weeks, the analgesic effects of lower doses will be restored (at least for a time).

Dependence

There are two types of dependence: physical and psychological dependence. There is much to recommend replacing physical dependence with the term 'neuroadaptation' (Edwards, cited in Jaffe, 1990); but this has not happened. For discussions with patients it is better to refer to psychological dependence as 'addiction'. This topic will be dealt with separately.

Physical dependence develops with the opioids and various other drugs. Physical dependence has developed when, if administration is suddenly ceased, the patient demonstrates an abstinence syndrome, or physical withdrawal. The common picture in opioid withdrawal includes muscle spasms, diarrhoea, and autonomic effects including tachycardia and piloerection (the source of the term, 'cold turkey'). These events can be both painful (not to mention the re-emergence of the pain that was the focus of treatment) and frightening.

Withdrawal effects are an expected response when drug use has altered physiology. This is clearly the case where tolerance has developed. Opioids suppress the production of endogenous endorphins, and on cessation of medication the body is left with less than normal levels of a physiological agent.

Withdrawal effects, albeit less dramatic, are associated with the withdrawal of the antiepileptics, venlafaxine, clonidine and many others.

Withdrawal effects can be avoided by tapering rather than suddenly ceasing medication.

Addiction (psychological dependence)

Addiction or psychological dependence refers to compulsive drug use, an overwhelming interest in securing a supply and the return to drug use after detoxification despite advice to the contrary. The term 'compulsive' is used here as it relates to 'compelled', which means to be forced or driven. Such behaviour causes the individual physical, psychological, or social harm.

Addiction is observed with drugs that have euphoric or other comforting psychological effects.

Addiction is suggested by aberrant drug-related behaviour, which includes increasing the amount of drug taken without medical direction, hoarding drugs 'in case' they are needed, obtaining drugs from different doctors and buying drugs illegally.

Many patients are reluctant to accept opioids because they fear addiction. Iatrogenic addiction can occur; however, the risk is low in the majority of patients, especially if clinicians are cautious and watch for aberrant drug-related behaviour. The risks are higher for those who are excessively impulsive or dependent. Where there is a history of drug abuse, treatment should proceed according to clear guidelines, preferably in collaboration with a clinician with special experience in addiction.

Many pain centres provide written information and require all patients to sign opioid treatment contracts (Bouckoms, 1996; Irving and Wallace, 1997). Information is provided regarding tolerance, dependence and addiction. Before receiving the patient must agree to adhere to directions, not to consult other doctors, hoard medication, or buy/sell drugs illegally, and not to use illegal drugs. Most contracts state that contravention of these conditions will result in discontinuation of the prescription of opioids.

Adverse effects

There is no organ toxicity, and thus no fatal adverse effects, when opioids are used according to directions. Respiratory arrest may occur in overdose.

Nausea and vomiting, constipation, sedation, pruritus, urinary retention, and sexual dysfunction are possible adverse effects, and their management has been detailed above.

Management principles

Opioids are not a panacea for chronic pain, and they all carry significant risks. Use in non-cancer pain is controversial by some accounts (Ward et al, 1993). However, Bouckoms et al (1992) reported the long-term treatment of large series of patients with non-cancer chronic pain in which 2/3 achieved effective pain relief. One-third demonstrated tolerance, physical dependency or drug abuse over a three-year period. Bennett (1999) recently stated that opiates are the most effective currently available treatment for most chronic pain states.

Opioids are considered to be more effective in non-neuropathic pain (Dellemijn, 1999). Nevertheless, beneficial effects are reported with neuropathic pain (Watson and Babul, 1998).

Opioids should only be considered when all other avenues for relief (non-opioid and co-analgesics) have been exhausted.

It is not possible to predict whether an opioid will be helpful in a particular case. This can only be determined through a clinical trial in which the dose is gradually escalated till pain relief occurs or intolerable adverse effects are experienced. Opioids differ from each other; so that if one fails to provide relief, it is worth trying others.

Brose and Spiegel (1992) caution against using inadequate doses. They advise that there is great individual variability, and that, for a particular drug, one patient may need five or six times the dose of another. However, Caraceni et al (2000) caution that failure to achieve at least partial analgesia with relatively low doses in the non-tolerant individual must raise doubts about the potential for opioid treatment.

Long-acting opioids taken twice daily (once daily if possible, depending on the case and the available preparations) are a fundamental of good opioid use in chronic pain. They allow the serum levels to be kept relatively constant. Fluctuations in serum levels lead to the frequent return of pain. The return of pain is frightening. Attempts to gain relief in these circumstances lead to excessive opioid use. With short-acting opioids fluctuations in serum levels are unavoidable. Thus short-acting opioids should not be used as the basis of chronic pain management. Further supporting this position is the fact that frequent ingestion of drugs followed by immediate relief and then the return of symptoms carries a greater risk of engendering addiction.

Even with stable serum opioid levels, patients may experience severe 'breakthrough' pain, sometimes for explicable reasons, such as increased activity, but often for no apparent reason.

The recommended regimen is a fixed dose of long-acting drug taken twice daily (once daily if this provides sufficient relief), with a limited supply of short-acting opioids to be taken for breakthrough pain. This arrangement provides a monitoring system. If the patient is needing an increased amount of short-acting opioid, and after consideration there is no evidence of aberrant drug behaviour, it is time to increase the dose of the load-bearing long-acting medication.

As was mentioned above, patients must be made aware of the potential risks and benefits. Many pain centres require the signature of an opioid management contract.

Improved physical and social functioning should be stressed. Pain relief should enable the patient to engage more actively with the world. Such changes in behaviour bring additional benefits.

Only one practitioner should prescribe the opioid for a particular patient. However, other clinicians should be involved in decisions to use very high doses, and when the treatment of patients with a history of drug abuse is being considered.

At each appointment the doctor should enquire into and record the degree of analgesia, adverse effects, physical and social activity and aberrant drug behaviour (preoccupation with drugs, hoarding, dose escalation, obtaining drugs from other sources).

Examples of opioids

A large range of opioid products are available. A selection is presented, using manufacturer recommendations: for complete details a pharmacology text should be consulted. Clinical practice may vary from these guidelines.

Chronic pain is generally managed using oral medication. Unless otherwise mentioned, the following details refer to the oral forms.

Long-acting drugs

These preparations form the backbone of opioid management of chronic pain.

Morphine sulphate in sustained-release form, marketed as *Kapanol*
Administered once, or at most twice, daily
Available as 10, 20, 50 and 100 mg capsules
Recommended starting dose: 20 mg twice daily, or 40 mg once daily
Conversion from other opioids depends on a variety of factors, and must be performed with caution. Oral morphine has a potency equivalent to oral oxycodone. When methadone is given regularly, it is 3–4 times more potent than oral morphine. Injected morphine has 3 times the potency of oral morphine.

Morphine sulphate in the sustained-release form, marketed as *MS Contin*
Administered twice daily

Available as 5, 10, 30, 60, 100, 200 mg tablets
Recommended starting dose: 30 mg twice daily.

Oxycodone hydrochloride in the controlled-release form, marketed as *Oxycontin*
Administered twice daily
Available as 10, 20, 40 and 80 mg tablets
Recommended starting dose: 10 mg twice daily

Fentanyl as a transdermal system (patch), marketed as *Durogesic*
A patch lasts 3 days.
Available as 25, 50, 75 and 100 micrograms per hour
Recommended starting dose, for opioid-naïve patients, 25 micrograms per hour. Peak concentrations of fentanyl occur between 24 to 72 hours after application. After the initial 72 hours, subsequent patches maintain a steady serum concentration. *Conversion from other opioids*: the fentanyl dose is based on the average daily use of opioids expressed as oral morphine equivalent, e.g. an equivalent of 135–224 mg of oral morphine per 24 hours is replaced with fentanyl 50 micrograms per hour. Tables are provided by the manufacturer. Individual titration will be necessary.

Short-acting opioid may be added for breakthrough pain and subsequently converted into this form of fentanyl.

This is a new and expensive product, and experience is limited.

Medium-acting drugs

Methadone marketed as *Physeptone*
Administered 3 times daily
Available as 5 and 10 mg tablets
Recommended starting dose: 10 mg 3 times daily
Methadone has less euphoric effect than the other opioids, and is less likely to be associated with addiction. It has an extremely long half life, which makes it valuable in preventing withdrawal in addicts, and can be given as a once-a-day dose. The analgesic half life, however, is much shorter; and for chronic pain relief purposes it must be taken more frequently. Inter-individual variability in the analgesic half life is a disadvantage, and many clinicians favour alternative, sustained-release products.

Tramadol marketed as *Tramal*
Administered three times daily
Available as 50 and 100 mg capsules
Recommended starting dose 50 mg three times daily. Manufacturer recommended maximum dose: 400 mg daily
This medication is difficult to classify. It has two actions (an opioid and a non-opioid action). It has a mu receptor affinity 6000 times less than morphine. There is no euphoria and there are no withdrawal or addiction problems. Thus some authorities list tramadol as a non-opioid drug. The primary analgesic effect appears to be through increasing the availability in the CNS of the neurotransmitters serotonin and norepinephrine. There are no serious adverse effects: nausea is the most common; others include somnolence and dizziness. It has been found effective in the pain of diabetic neuropathy (Harati et al, 1998), pain and allodynia in polyneuropathy (Sindrup et al, 1999) and chronic low back pain (Schnitzer et al, 2000).

Short-acting drugs

In chronic pain management, these preparations are best reserved for breakthrough pain:

Morphine sulphate immediate-release preparation, marketed as *Anamorph* (and others)
Administered on an as-needed basis.
Available as 30 mg tablets.
Onset is rapid, at 15–20 minutes. Duration of action is 3–4 hours.

Codeine phosphate marketed as *Codeine phosphate (and others)*
Administered on an as-needed basis.
Available as 30 mg tablet.
This is a weak opioid. It has a quicker onset and a shorter duration than morphine. In some products it is in combination with paracetamol, aspirin or acetaminophen.

Oxycodone hydrochloride immediate-release preparation, marketed as *Endone* Administered on an as-needed basis. Available as 5 mg tablet.

Non-steroidal anti-inflammatory drugs (NSAIDs) (cyclooxygenase inhibitors)

The NSAIDs are antipyretic, and their anti-inflammatory action provides useful analgesic effects. The prostaglandins induce inflammation and sensitize primary afferent nerves. The NSAIDs inhibit the enzyme cyclooxygenase (COX), thereby reducing the production of prostaglandins. The NSAIDs probably also have central analgesic effects.

COX exists in at least two physiological forms (COX-1 and COX-2). Most currently available NSAIDs are non-specific inhibitors of both isoforms. COX-1 inhibition is associated with GI (and renal) toxicity, while COX-2 inhibition reduces inflammation and pain.

Adverse effects

Adverse effects are related to COX inhibition. As was stated above, GI symptoms occur in 10% of patients treated. Ulcers and haemorrhage may occur without warning. When there are previous symptoms or risk factors, gastric protection (a prostaglandin analogue, a proton pump inhibitor or a

histamine H_2 receptor antagonist) should be considered. Selective COX-2 inhibiting NSAIDs have a clear advantage.

Inhibition of platelet aggregation is a serious concern, particularly for patients with pre-existing bleeding problems, those receiving anticoagulant therapy and the medically frail.

Nephrotoxicity from NSAIDs is rare in the healthy patient. However, the risk is increased in patients with renal disease, volume depletion, congestive heart failure or cirrhosis.

Exacerbation of bronchospasm can occur, and may cause coughing at night. Hypersensitivity reactions are rare: they range from mild cutaneous eruptions to life-threatening anaphylaxis.

An interaction with lithium has been claimed. However, to this point the author has been able to find only case reports regarding piroxicam and dicolfenac raising the serum level of lithium. Sulindac may have a minimal effect.

Monitoring may include tests for occult faecal blood, haemoglobin level and renal and hepatic function. Endoscopy is indicated when GI symptoms are experienced.

Management principles

NSAIDs are used for mild to moderate pain, especially pain secondary to an inflammatory component. They have a ceiling effect. There is individual variation between patients with respect to the optimal drug and dose. Serial trials of different NSAIDs, working up to maximal doses, are justified. They are generally believed to be less effective in neuropathic pain, but they may offer some relief in this situation. They enhance opioid analgesia and reduce the opioid requirement.

Selective COX-2 inhibitors are becoming available (celecoxib, rofecoxib and nimesulide) and are recommended where they can be afforded.

Treatment should commence at a low dose, and can be increased at the end of one week if analgesia is not achieved. The following list is composed from manufacturers' product information, supplemented from papers and leading texts. Some manufacturers do not state that their medications should be taken with food. Owing to the high prevalence of GI symptoms, however, this would be sensible advice.

Examples of NSAIDs

A large range of NSAID products are available. A selection is presented, using manufacturer recommendations: for complete details a pharmacology text should be consulted. Clinical practice may vary from these guidelines.

Selective COX-2 inhibitor
Celecoxib
Administered once or twice daily
Available as 100 and 200 mg capsules
Recommended starting dose: 100 mg once daily
Maximum dose: 200 mg twice daily

Non-selective COX inhibitors – arranged in order of increasing frequency of administration

Ketoprofen marketed in slow release form as *Orudis*
Administered once daily
Available as 100 and 200 mg capsules
Recommended starting dose: 100 mg daily
Maximum dose 300 mg daily (Insel, 1990)

Piroxicam
Administered once a day
Available as 10 and 20 mg capsules
Recommended starting dose: 10 mg once daily
Maximum dose limit is not available.
Good response has been obtained with 20 mg daily.

Sulindac
Administered once (at night) or twice daily with food or fluid
Available as 100 and 200 mg tablets
Recommended starting dose: 100 mg daily
Maximum dose: 400 mg daily

Diflunisal

Administered twice daily

Available as 250 and 500 mg tablets

Recommended starting dose: 500 mg twice daily

Maximum dose: 2000 mg daily

Naproxen

Administered twice a day

Available as 250 and 500 mg tablets

Recommended starting dose: 250 mg twice daily

Maximum dose: 3200 mg daily (Insel, 1990)

Diclofenac

Administered three or four times daily: swallow with liquid

Available as 25 mg and 50 mg tablets

Recommended starting dose: 50 mg twice daily

Maximum dose: 200 mg daily

Ibuprofen

Administered three to six times daily with food or fluid

Available as 400 mg tablet

Recommended starting dose: 1200–1600 mg daily

Maximum dose: 2400 mg daily

Antidepressants

The antidepressants, particularly the tricyclic antidepressants (TCAs), have an important place in the management of chronic pain (McQuay and Moore, 1998). This analgesic effect is not due to antidepressant effects, although relieving any existing depression makes the patient more able to tolerate pain.

A protective mechanism in the CNS works to reduce pain experienced by the organism. Norepinephrine and serotonin pathways descend in the dorsal column to the dorsal horns, where they inhibit nociceptor input into the second-order neurones. Certain antidepressants significantly increase this dorsal horn inhibition.

Other actions of the TCAs that potentially contribute to the analgesic effects are the usually undesired features of alpha-1 and NMDA blockade. The TCAs also have an antihistamine action that may play an analgesic role. Bouckoms (1996) suggested that their ability to upregulate mesolimbic dopamine may be important.

Fishbain (2000) conducted an evidence-based review and concluded that antidepressants have an analgesic effect, which was particularly evident in neuropathic pain. Sindrup and Jensen (2000), using different statistical methodology, compared the drugs used for pain in polyneuropathy and concluded that TCAs remain the drugs of first choice. Kanazi et al (2000) found TCAs to be as effective as the other existing treatments of postherpetic neuralgia. Fishbain (2000) found TCAs were effective in some specific pain syndromes, including chronic low back pain, osteoarthritis, rheumatoid arthritis, fibromyalgia and ulcer healing. O'Malley et al (1999) and Arnold et al (2000) also found TCAs to be valuable in the treatment of fibromyalgia.

The drugs that increase both norepinephrine and serotonin in the synaptic cleft are effective in pain. The SSRIs have much less analgesic effect (O'Malley et al, 1999; Arnold et al, 2000; Fishbain, 2000). Venlafaxine is a novel serotonin and norepinephrine reuptake inhibitor that, while safer in overdose, is similar in action to the TCAs at high dose. It has not yet been studied as an analgesic, but it may have a place in migraine and tension headache prophylaxis (Adelman et al, 2000).

The monoamine oxidase inhibitors (MAOIs) may have some analgesic effects, but they have not been studied and are little used in the field. There is a potentially dangerous interaction of MAOIs and pethidine. The reversible MAOI, moclobemide, was found to ease pain in fibromyalgia, but overall, it was not helpful, as sleep was not improved (Hannonen et al, 1998).

The analgesic effects of the TCAs usually commence at lower doses than are commonly employed for the treatment of depression. These effects usually occur in less than a week, and where pain and depression coexist, the pain responds first. TCAs can be commenced at low doses of 25 mg *nocte* and increased over several weeks. Analgesic effects are dose-dependent, and doses of 150 mg amitriptyline (Max et al, 1987) and beyond have been used with good effect.

As was mentioned above, the sedative effect of tertiary amine TCAs (amitriptyline, imipramine) may be beneficial when there are sleep problems. Where daytime sedation remains a problem, the secondary amines should be offered (nortriptyline, desipramine). Very slow TCA metabolism leading to excessive side-effects results from the absence of certain liver enzymes in about 5% of people.

Plasma levels of TCAs may be determined. This may be useful where non compliance or very rapid or slow metabolism are suspected. Levels may also serve as legal protection if high doses are employed.

Adverse effects

The adverse effects of sedation, constipation, orthostatic hypotension, dry mouth, blurred vision, urinary retention and sexual dysfunction have been discussed above. The TCAs are relatively contraindicated for patients with significant cardiac arrhythmia, prostatic hypertrophy or narrow angle glaucoma due to anticholinergic actions. They may cause fatal cardiac conduction problems in overdose.

Selection of antidepressants

A large range of antidepressant products are available. A selection is presented, using manufacturer recommendations: for complete details, a pharmacology text should be consulted. Clinical practice may vary from these guidelines.

TCAs

Amitriptyline
Administered as a single dose at night or divided doses through the day
Available as 10, 25 and 50 mg tablets
Recommended starting dose: 25 mg
Maximum dose: 300 mg daily

Nortriptyline
Administered as a single dose at night or divided doses through the day
Available as 10 and 25 mg tablets
Recommended stating dose 25 mg
Maximum dose: 100 mg daily*
Nortriptyline is a metabolite, and less sedating than amitriptyline.

Desipramine
Administered in divided doses through the day
Available as 25 mg tablets
Recommended stating dose: 25 mg *mane*
Maximum dose: 200 mg*
Desipramine is a metabolite of imipramine. It

is the least sedating TCA, and in some patients may even have a stimulating effect.

* Manufacturer recommendations. In clinical practice these doses have been exceeded using serum concentration guidelines.

SSRIs

Fluoxetine
Administered in the morning, increasing to twice daily if necessary
Available as 20 mg capsules
Recommended starting dose: 20 mg
Maximum dose: 80 mg daily

Other SSRI preparations are commonly used in the treatment of depression (fluvoxamine, sertraline, paroxetine, citalopram). Evidence suggests they are equally effective in depression, but are poor analgesics.

Anticonvulsants

The anticonvulsants are a group of unrelated drugs with generally similar, but different, actions, adverse effects and clinical applications. Members have a role in the management of neuropathic pain and headache prophylaxis (see the chapter on headache).

Neuropathic pain may have many pathophysiologic features. One may be ectopic firing of damaged peripheral neurones secondary to instability of sodium channels. Another is purported to be central sensitivity to nociception mediated by activation of N-methyl-D-aspartate (NMDA) receptors. These receptors are activated by inflow of calcium ions into the post-synaptic dorsal horn cells. The usefulness of the anticonvulsants in neuropathic pain may arise from ability to influence these or other processes, including modulation of gamma-aminobutyric acid (GABA).

Carbamazepine blocks both sodium and calcium channels. Valproate blocks sodium channels and increases GABA levels. Gabapentin blocks both sodium and calcium channels and increases GABA levels. Our knowledge is preliminary, however, and these may not be the important pharmacological effects.

Carbamazepine (Blom, 1962) and valproate (Raftery, 1979) have been used in the treatment of neuropathic pain for decades. Gabapentin has been shown effective in postherpetic neuralgia (Rowbotham et al, 1998) and painful diabetic neuropathy (Backonja et al, 1998).

A review (Wiffen et al, 2000) looking at the efficacy and adverse effects of the anticonvulsants, however, concluded that, in chronic pain syndromes other than trigeminal neuralgia, the anticonvulsants should be withheld until other interventions have been tried. The authors also found that the evidence suggested that gabapentin is not superior to carbamazepine.

Other reviews focusing on gabapentin (Laird and Gidal, 2000; Ross, 2000; Tremont-Lukats et al, 2000) have concluded that this drug has an analgesic effect in neuropathic pain, and is better tolerated than the older antidepressants. Laird and Gidal (2000) and Termont-Lukats et al (2000) found that gabapentin should be the drug of first choice in the treatment of neuropathic pain. Laird and Gidal (2000) added that the expense of this drug was a disincentive to use.

Caraceni et al (2000) point out that future studies may show the anticonvulsants to be as non-specific as the TCAs. They point out that patients may have markedly different responses to drugs, and hence sequential trials of the anticonvulsants are justified.

Adverse effects

As the anticonvulsants are chemically unrelated they have different constellations of adverse effects. They all have effects on neural tissue, and therefore can be expected to cause lethargy, somnolence, dizziness, ataxia and tremor. This is less severe in gabapentin. They can all cause nausea, vomiting and diarrhoea, again, less severely with gabapentin.

Additional non-serious adverse effects include fluid retention and rash/itch with carbamazepine, weight gain and hair loss with valproate and non-pitting oedema with gabapentin. (The hair loss associated with valproate is eminently treatable with zinc supplementation.)

Rare life-threatening idiosyncratic reactions are similar for carbamazepine and valproate, and include agranulocytosis, Stevens–Johnson syndrome, aplastic anaemia, thrombocytopenia, hepatic failure, dermatitis, serum sickness and pancreatitis. Gabapentin does not have severe adverse effects.

Management principles

Drugs should be started at low levels and gradually increased to reduce the occurrence of adverse effects. The serum levels used in epilepsy do not apply in pain management (Irving and Wallace, 1997) and the dose is determined by balancing therapeutic response and adverse effects. Serum levels may provide legal protection for the clinician when high doses are used.

Liver function tests (LFTs) and full blood count (FBC) are taken at baseline. Except for gabapentin (which is not metabolized in the liver) these are repeated monthly for three months, and then three- to six-monthly.

Examples of anticonvulsants

A large range of anticonvulsants is available. A selection is presented, using manufacturer recommendations: for complete details, a pharmacology text should be consulted. The newer anticonvulsants, lamotrigine and

tropiramate, have yet to be evaluated as analgesics. Clinical practice may vary from these guidelines.

Carbamazepine

Administered 3 to 4 times daily for conventional tablets and liquid; twice daily for the controlled-release tablets; swallow during or after meals with fluid.

Available as 100 and 200 mg conventional tablets; liquid 100 mg/5 ml; 200 and 400 mg controlled-release tablets

Starting dose (trigeminal neuralgia): 200–400 mg daily

Maximal dose: 1200 mg daily

Valproate

Administered twice daily

Available as 100, 200, 500 mg tablets and syrup and sugar-free liquid 200 mg/5 ml

Starting dose: 600 mg daily

Maximum dose: 2500 mg daily

Gabapentin

Administered three times daily

Available as 300 and 400 mg capsules

Starting dose 300 mg on day 1, 600 mg on day 2, 900 mg on day 3. To minimize adverse effects, the day 1 dose should be given at bedtime.

Maximum dose: 2400 mg daily (reports in the literature to 3600 mg daily).

Local anaesthetic/ antiarrhythmic agents (sodium channel blockers)

These drugs have been classified both as local anaesthetics and as antiarrhythmic agents, these labels perhaps reflecting the backgrounds of different authors. While they have other actions, the most important action appears to be sodium channel blockade. This is an action they share with the anticonvulsants.

These agents are applied systemically (intravenously or orally). A sodium channel blocker suppresses abnormal activity in damaged neurones, without blocking normal nerve conduction. Thus they have been used in neuropathic pain. However, central effects have also been postulated, and intravenous lignocaine has been found useful for intractable headache.

Intravenous lignocaine has also been found effective in various conditions in reviews of the treatment of general neuropathic pain (Mao and Chen, 2000; Kalso et al, 1998; Kingery, 1997) and postherpetic neuralgia (Bonezzi and Demartini, 1999). A Japanese report indicated a favourable response in the painful neuropathy of multiple sclerosis (Sakurai and Kanazawa, 1999). The effect of an infusion may last many months. A trial of intravenous lignocaine is appropriate for patients with neuropathic pain who are otherwise healthy.

Mexiletine is structurally related to lignocaine. It is available as an oral preparation and has been used in the treatment of painful neuropathy. Reviews found little support for mexiletine in the treatment of chronic pain (Kalso et al, 1998) and painful diabetic neuropathy (Jarvis and Coukell, 1998), but concluded that the drug may have a place when other treatments have failed. More recently, no benefit was determined in the treatment of HIV-related painful peripheral neuropathy (Kemper et al, 1998) or neuropathic pain with prominent allodynia (Wallace et al, 2000). This evidence indicates that mexiletine is, at best, a second-line drug in the treatment of neuropathic pain.

Management principles

Patients with significant heart disease should not receive intravenous lignocaine. Those who could be at risk should obtain a cardiology consultation.

A lignocaine infusion is 1–5 mg/kg administered over 20–30 minutes (Baranowski et al, 1999). As dose-dependent effects have been reported, treatment should commence within the lower level of the range. If the low-dose infusion is unsuccessful, a higher dose infusion should be considered Constant ECG and blood pressure monitoring is necessary, and resuscitative equipment and drugs, including oxygen, should be immediately available.

Similarly, mexiletine should be commenced when the risk of cardiac complications has been appropriately considered. The starting dose should be low, and increases should be gradual. The serum levels used in cardiology are not relevant when the drug is used for pain relief.

Adverse effects

The adverse effects of lignocaine and mexiletine are similar, but the emphasis is different, reflecting the different modes of administration. They include lightheadedness, drowsiness, apprehension, euphoria, tinnitus, blurred vision, nystagmus, gastrointestinal symptoms, vomiting, twitching tremors, disorientation, confusion, dyspnoea, slurred speech, convulsions, unconsciousness, respiratory arrest, hypotension, arrhythmia, heart block, bradycardia, cardiac arrest and allergic skin reactions.

Mexiletine causes more gastric discomfort, vomiting, unpleasant taste and oesophageal ulceration (if a capsule is lodged in the oesophagus because inadequate liquid has been swallowed). Transient tachycardia and palpitations but not serious cardiac arrhythmias have been reported in pain studies (Jarvis and Coukell, 1998; Kemper et al, 1998; Wallace et al, 2000).

Selection of local anaesthetic/antiarrhythmic agents

The following is derived from manufacturer recommendations and leading research papers. For complete details a pharmacology text should be consulted. Clinical practice may vary from these guidelines.

Lignocaine
Administered by elective intravenous infusion
Available as 10 mg/ml, in 10 ml ampoules, and 20 mg/ml, in 5 ml ampoules
Starting dose at the low level of the range 1–5 mg/kg, over 20–30 minutes.
Maximal dose: 5 mg/kg.

Mexiletine
Administered three times daily
Available as 50 and 200 mg capsules
Starting dose: 50 mg three times daily, increasing by 50 mg daily
Maximum dose: 10 mg/kg daily, or 900 mg, whichever is the lower.

Alpha-1 antagonists and alpha-2 agonists

Sympathetically maintained pain (SMP) is a purported form of neuropathic pain that is sustained by efferent activity in the sympathetic nervous system. The most severe type is complex regional pain syndrome (CRPS), or causalgia. This provides a theoretical basis for specific use of alpha-1 antagonists and alpha-2 agonists. The picture is not yet clear, however, and some (Caraceni et al, 2000) consider the alpha-2 agonists to be non-specific analgesics.

Peripheral nerve terminals support alpha-1 receptors. Stimulation of these receptors on damaged nerves by ephedrine from sympathetic nerve terminals may be a cause of pain. Preganglionic nerves have pre-synaptic alpha-2 receptors. Stimulation of these receptors reduces the release of ephedrine into the ganglionic synapse and, thereby, activity in the post-ganglionic cell and release of ephedrine on to the peripheral nerve terminal. Thus a chemical sympathectomy can be achieved by alpha-2 agonistic activity on the preganglionic cell and alpha-1 antagonism of target receptors.

Both types of drugs have neurological effects; thus any analgesic effect may be mediated partially or wholly by central actions.

While the theory is attractive, oral and transdermal alpha-1 antagonists and alpha-2 agonists have not achieved clinical prominence. The alpha-1 antagonist, phenoxybenzamine, has been used with some success in CRPS (Ghostine et al, 1984; Muizelaar et al, 1997). The alpha-2 agonist, clonidine, administered transdermally has been useful for a small proportion of patients with postherpetic neuralgia (Byas-Smith et al, 1995). They have significant adverse effects

profiles, and, with their modest efficacy, they are generally thought to be drugs of second choice.

Some evidence suggests clonidine may be combined with opioids, when tolerance to opioids has developed (Bouckoms, 1996). Clonidine has been used in combination with other analgesics administered by intraspinal injection.

Doctors with special experience use phentolamine, an alpha-1 and alpha-2 blocker, to determine whether oral treatment is likely to provide relief. Phentolamine, 0.5–1.0 mg/kg, is infused intravenously over 30 minutes. Pain relief with this procedure supports a trial of oral medication. This test is not universally employed, however, and a trial of oral medication will reveal whether it offers benefits.

Adverse effects

The adverse effects of these drugs can be minimized by starting with low doses and increasing gradually, and many subside over two to three weeks. Both types of drug may cause hypotension, drowsiness, nausea and vomiting.

Clonidine may cause sinus bradycardia and atrioventricular block; phenoxybenzamine may cause tachycardia.

These drugs are also associated with a wide range of less common effects, including nasal congestion, dry mouth, hair loss, blurred vision, diarrhoea, constipation, depression, psychotic symptoms, pruritus, rash, impotence, fever and diaphoresis (this is not an exhaustive list).

In two studies of phenoxybenzamine for CRPS (Ghostine et al, 1984; Muizelaar et al, 1997), with a total of 99 patients, the adverse effects were considered to be minimal and transient.

Examples of alpha-1 antagonists and alpha-2 agonists

A small range of oral alpha-1 antagonists is available; only one is presented. For complete details a pharmacology text should be consulted. Clinical practice may vary from these guidelines.

Alpha-1 antagonist
Phenoxybenzamine
Administered twice daily
Available 10 mg capsules
Starting dose: 10 mg twice daily. Increase by 10 mg every other day
Maximum dose: 60 mg daily

Phentolamine
Administered as a test of responsiveness of pain to alpha antagonism
Available 10 mg/1 ml.

Alpha-2 agonist
Clonidine
Administered twice daily
Available as 100 and 150 microgram tablets
Starting dose: 50 micrograms twice daily.
Increase by 50 micrograms, every other day
Maximum dose: 600 micrograms

NMDA receptor antagonists

Recent advances in our knowledge of the N-methyl-D-aspartate (NMDA) and related receptors appear to set the stage for important developments in the management of chronic pain. We await the ready availability of proven non-toxic, potent NMDA receptor blockers.

Dorsal horn cells, which process nociceptive input, display, along with a range of others, mu opioid and NMDA receptors. Part of the basis of the centrally mediated hyperalgesia that occurs in chronic pain states is the sensitization of NMDA receptors, as a consequence of continuous input from the periphery. The mu opioid and NMDA receptors share certain intracellular processes such that the NMDA receptor may also become progressively sensitized as a result of progressive opioid administration. Theory suggests that NMDA receptor blockers will have analgesic properties, that hyperalgesia and opioid tolerance will occur together, and that NMDA blockade will prevent/reverse opioid tolerance. There are consistent experimental findings (Mao et al, 1995; Price et al, 2000).

As was pointed out above, some of the analgesic effects of the anticonvulsants may derive from NMDA blockade. A collection of other blockers is being researched as analgesics (ketamine, dextromethorphan, amantadine), but none have become routine treatment.

The effects of oral ketamine on chronic neuropathic pain were retrospectively examined in 21 patients (Enarson et al, 1999). Only three obtained substantial benefits. Better results may be possible using the intravenous route (Galer et al, 1993). A review (Weinbroun et al, 2000) of the clinical benefits of dextromethorphan in chronic pain found unsatisfactory pain relief. The authors also examined the evidence for dextromethorphan in acute pain, and found an attenuation of pain, with tolerable adverse effects. Intravenous amantadine has been shown to be effective in surgical neuropathic pain (Pud et al, 1998), but not in sciatica (Medrik-Goldberg et al, 1999).

Exciting evidence suggests that ketamine (Mercadante et al, 2000) and dextromethorphan (Price et al, 2000) increase the analgesic effects of morphine. These studies suggest a capacity to reduce tolerance to morphine that is considered probable. Such a capacity would have wide application within pain management and potentially in addiction medicine.

Adverse effects

The NMDA receptor blockers are a disparate group of drugs; therefore they have different constellations of adverse effects. Mention has been made of the adverse effects of the anticonvulsants.

Ketamine has a wide range of adverse effects. Heart rate and blood pressure have been both raised and lowered. Arrhythmia has occurred. Respiration is frequently stimulated; however, respiratory depression, laryngospasm and obstruction may occur. Diplopia and nystagmus have been noted. Hallucinations and delirium occur. (These have been thought to occur only at anaesthetic doses. However, Mercadante et al (2000) report them at sub-anaesthetic doses.) Tonic and clonic movements, anorexia, nausea, vomiting and morbiliform rash have been reported.

Selection of NMDA blocking drugs

Ketamine is the only NMDA blocking drug (apart from the anticonvulsants) that is commercially available in a form that might be useful in chronic pain management. Dextromethorphan is available as an antitussive syrup and amantadine is available as a capsule (and is used as an antiviral and antiparkinsonian agent).

Ketamine
Available as ampoules and vials, 200 mg (base)/2 ml
Oral administration: Enarson et al (1999) started at 100 mg daily in divided doses and

increased by 40 mg daily till relief or till symptoms became intolerable. The highest dose they used was 500 mg daily.

Intravenous administration: Galer et al (1993) provided 5 mg/kg/hour for 60 to 90 minutes.

GABA-potentiators (benzodiazepine receptor agonists/anxiolytics)

Gamma-amino-butyric acid (GABA) is an abundant neurotransmitter. GABA A receptors are the gatekeepers of chloride channels. Stimulation of the receptor opens the channel and inhibits the neurone. There is a specific benzodiazepine receptor on the GABA A receptor. When the benzodiazepine receptor is occupied, GABA has a greater effect, causing wider opening of the chloride channel and greater neuronal inhibition than when the benzodiazepine receptor is unoccupied.

Clonazepam may be grouped with the anticonvulsants, as this is a clinical role, but its action is distinct and there is some evidence for use in neuropathic pain (Reddy and Patt, 1994; Bartusch et al, 1996).

Tolerance and withdrawal may develop with the benzodiazepines, which can further complicate the management of difficult cases. These drugs have a place in the management of anxiety and, to some extent, muscle spasm. With the possible exception of clonazepam in neuropathic pain, these drugs do not have a place as analgesics.

Monoamine receptor blockers (antipsychotics)

Blockers of combinations of dopamine and serotonin (along with other) receptors are used in the management of psychosis. These medications have a place when there is comorbid psychosis or delirium. Prochlorperazine has a place in the treatment of nausea. There is little evidence to support claims that these drugs have useful analgesic effects (Patt et al, 1994).

Histamine receptor blockers (antihistamines)

Histamine receptors are found throughout the nervous system. The mechanism by which analgesia may be achieved remains theoretical (Galeotti et al, 1999). There is some evidence that diphenhydramine, hydroxyzine, orphenadrine and pyrilamine have analgesic effects (Rumore and Schlichting, 1986). The antihistamines have been used in combination, in the hope of augmenting known analgesics.

Sedation is a complication of most of these drugs, and, as there is no strong evidence of analgesic benefit, they are better considered a last choice strategy.

Sympathomimetic agents (stimulants)

Dextroamphetamine, methylphenidate and caffeine, along with other actions, stimulate adrenoreceptors. There is some evidence that these agents possess intrinsic analgesic properties; but this is minor and does not justify use. There is also evidence that the amphetamines can enhance opioids (Dalal and Melzack, 1998). Caffeine has been used to potentiate the effects of ibuprofen in tension-type headache (Diamond et al, 2000).

The main place of the stimulants in pain medicine is in the management of opioid-induced fatigue and insomnia (Corey et al, 1999). This is an infrequent use in chronic non-cancer pain. Owing to their adverse effects, addiction and psychosis, these drugs are best avoided whenever possible.

References

Adelman L, Adelman J, Von Seggern R, Mannix L. Venlafaxine extended release (XR) for the prophylaxis of migraine and tension-type headache: A retrospective study in a clinical setting. *Headache* 2000; 40: 572–80.

Arnold L, Keck P, Welge J. Antidepressant treatment of fibromyalgia. A meta-analysis and review. *Psychosomatics* 2000; 41: 104–13.

Backonja M, Beydoun A, Edwards K, et al. Gabapentin for the symptomatic treatment of painful neuropathy in patients with diabetes mellitus: a randomized controlled trial. *Journal of the American Medical Association* 1998; 280: 1831–6.

Baranowski A, De Courcey J, Bonello E. A trial of intravenous lidocaine on the pain and allodynia of postherpetic neuralgia. *Journal of Pain and Symptom Management* 1999; 17: 429–33.

Bartusch S, Sanders B, D'Alessio J, Jernigan J. Clonazepam for the treatment of lancinating phantom limb pain. *Clinical Journal of Pain* 1996; 12: 59–62.

Bennett R. Emerging concepts in the neurobiology of chronic pain: evidence of abnormal sensory processing in fibromyalgia. *Mayo Clinic Proceedings* 1999; 74: 385–98.

Blom S. Trigeminal neuralgia: its treatment with a new anticonvulsant drug (G32883). *Lancet* 1962; 1: 839–40.

Bonezzi C, Demartini L. Treatment options in postherpetic neuralgia. *Acta Neurologica Scandinavica* Suppl 1999; 173: 25–35.

Bouckoms A. Chronic pain: neuropsychopharmacology and adjunctive psychiatric treatment. In: Rundell J, Wise M (eds) *Textbook of Consultation-Liaison Psychiatry*. American Psychiatric Press, Washington, DC, 1996; 1007–36.

Bouckoms A, Masand P, Murray G, et al. Non-malignant pain treated with long term oral narcotics. *Annals of Clinical Psychiatry* 1992; 4: 185–92.

Brescia J, Portenoy R, Ryan M, et al. Pain, opioid use and survival in hospitalized patients with advanced cancer. *Journal of Clinical Oncology* 1992; 10: 149–55.

Brose W, Spiegel D. Neuropsychiatric aspects of pain management. In: Yudofsky S and Hales R (eds) *The American Psychiatric Textbook of Neuropsychiatry*, 2nd edn. American Psychiatric Press, Washington, DC, 1992; 245–75.

Byas-Smith M, Max M, Muir H, Kingman A. Transdermal clonidine compared to placebo in painful diabetic neuropathy using a two-staged 'enriched enrollment' design. *Pain* 1995; 60: 67–74.

Caraceni A, Cheville A, Portenoy R. Pain management: pharmacological and nonpharmacological treatments. In: Massie MJ (ed) *Pain: What Psychiatrists Need to Know* (Review of Psychiatry Series, Vol. 19, No 2; Oldham J and Riba M, series eds). American Psychiatric Press, Washington, DC, 2000; 23–88.

Corey P, Heck A, Weathermon R. Amphetamine to counteract opioid-induced sedation. *Annals of Pharmacotherapy* 1999; 33: 1362–6.

Dalal S, Melzack R. Potentiation of opioid analgesia by psychostimulant drugs: a review. *Journal of Pain and Symptom Management* 1998; 16: 245–53.

Dellemijn P. Are opioids effective in relieving neuropathic pain? *Pain* 1999; 80: 453–62.

Diamond S, Balm T, Freitag F. Ibuprofen plus caffeine in the treatment of tension-type headache. *Clinics in Pharmacological Therapy* 2000; 68: 312–19.

Enarson M, Hays H, Woodroffe M. Clinical experience with oral ketamine. *Journal of Pain and Symptom Management* 1999; 17: 384–6.

Fishbain D. Evidence-based data on pain relief with antidepressants. *Annals of Medicine* 2000; 32: 305–16.

Galer B, Miller K, Rowbotham M. Response to intravenous lidocaine infusion differs based on clinical diagnosis and site of nervous system injury. *Neurology* 1993; 43: 1233–5.

Galeotti N, Ghelardini C, Bartolini A. The role of potassium channels in antihistamine analgesia. *Neuropharmacology* 1999; 38: 1893–901.

Ghostine S, Comair Y, Turner D, Kassell N, Azar C. Phenoxybenzamine in the treatment of causalgia. Report of 40 cases. *Journal of Neurosurgery* 1984; 60: 1263–8.

Grebb J. General principles of psychopharmacology. In: Kaplan H, Sadock B (eds) *Comprehensive Textbook of Psychiatry*, 6th edn. Williams & Wilkins, Baltimore, MD, 1995; 1895–909.

Hannonen P, Milminiemi K, Yli-Kerttula U, Isomeri R, Roponen P. A randomized, double-blind, placebo-controlled study of moclobemide and amitriptyline in the treatment of fibromyalgia in females without psychiatric disorder. *British Journal of Rheumatology* 1998; 1279–86.

Harati Y, Gooch C, Swenson M, Edelman S, Greene D, Raskin P, Donofrio P, Cornblath D, Sachdeo R, Siu C, Kamin M. Double-blind randomized trial of tramadol for the treatment of the pain of diabetic neuropathy. *Neurology* 1998; 50: 1842–6.

Insel P. Analgesic-antipyretics and antiinflammatory agents; drugs employed in the treatment of rheumatoid arthritis and gout. In: Gilman A, Rall T, Nies A, Taylor P (eds) *The Pharmacological Basis of Therapeutics*, 8th edn. Pergamon Press, New York, 1990; 638–81.

Irving G, Wallace M. *Pain Management for the Practicing Physician*. Churchill Livingstone, Philadelphia, 1997.

Jaffe J. Drug addiction and drug abuse. In: Gilman A, Rall T, Nies A, Taylor P (eds) *The Pharmacological Basis of Therapeutics*, 8th edn. Pergamon Press, New York, 1990; 522–30.

Jarvis B, Coukell A. Mexiletine. A review of its therapeutic use in painful diabetic neuropathy. *Drugs* 1998; 56: 691–707.

Kalso E, Tramer M, McQuay H, Moore R. Systematic local-anaesthetic-type drugs in chronic pain: a systematic review. *European Journal of Pain* 1998; 2: 3–14.

Kanazi G, Johnson R, Dworkin R. Treatment of postherpetic neuralgia. *Drugs* 2000; 59: 1113–26.

Kemper C, Kent G, Burton S, Deresinski S.

Mexiletine for HIV-infected patients with painful peripheral neuropathy: a double-blind, placebo-controlled, crossover treatment trial. *Journal of Acquired Immune Deficiency Syndrome and Human Retrovirology* 1998; 19: 367–72.

Kingery W. A critical review of controlled clinical trials for peripheral neuropathic pain and complex regional pain syndrome. *Pain* 1997; 73: 123–39.

Labbate L, Pollack M. Treatment of fluoxetine-induced sexual dysfunction with bupropion: a case report. *Annals of Clinical Psychiatry* 1994; 6: 13–15.

Laird M, Gidal B. Use of gabapentin in the treatment of neuropathic pain. *Annals Pharmacotherapy* 2000; 34: 802–7.

Mao J, Chen L. Systemic lidocaine for neuropathic pain relief. *Pain* 2000; 87: 7–17.

Mao J, Price D, Mayer D. Mechanisms of hyperalgesia and morphine tolerance: a current view of their possible interactions. *Pain* 1995; 62: 259–74.

Max M, Culnane M, Schafer S, Gracely R, Walther D, Smoller B, Dubner R. Amitriptyline relieves diabetic neuropathy pain in patients with normal or depressed mood. *Neurology* 1987; 37: 589–96.

McQuay H, Moore A. *An Evidence-Based Resource for Pain Relief.* Oxford, Oxford University Press, 1998.

Medrik-Goldberg T, Lifschitz D, Pud D, Adler R, Eisenberg E. Intravenous lidocaine, amantadine, and placebo in the treatment of sciatica: a double-blind, randomized, controlled study. *Regional Anesthesia and Pain Medicine* 1999; 24: 534–40.

Mercadante S, Arcuri E, Tirelli W, Casuccio A. Analgesic effects of intravenous ketamine in cancer patients or on morphine therapy. A randomized, controlled, double-blind, crossover, double-dose study. *Journal of Pain and Symptom Management* 2000; 20: 246–52.

Muizelaar J, Kleyer M, Hertogs I, DeLange D. Complex regional pain syndrome (reflex sympathetic dystrophy and causalgia): management with the calcium channel blocker nifedipine and/or the alpha-sympathetic blocker phenoxybenzamine in 59 patients. *Clinical Neurology and Neurosurgery* 1997; 99: 26–30.

O'Malley P, Jackson J, Santoro J, Tomkins G, Balden E, Krownke K. Antidepressant therapy for unexplained symptoms and symptom syndromes. *Journal of Family Practice* 1999; 48: 980–90.

Patt R, Proper G, Reddy S. The neuroleptics as adjuvant analgesics. *Journal of Pain and Symptom Management* 1994; 9: 446–53.

Pud D, Eisenberg E, Spitzer A, Adler R, Fried G, Yarnitsky D. The NMDA receptor antagonist reduces surgical neuropathic pain in cancer patients: a double blind, randomized, placebo controlled trial. *Pain* 1998; 75: 349–54.

Price D, Mayer D, Mao J. NMDA-receptor and opioid receptor interactions as related to analgesia and tolerance. *Journal of Pain and Symptom Management* 2000; 19: S7–11.

Raftery H. The management of post herpetic pain using sodium valproate and amitriptyline. *Irish Medical Journal* 1979; 72: 399–401.

Reddy S, Patt R. The benzodiazepines as adjuvant analgesics. *Journal of Pain and Symptom Management* 1994; 9: 510–14.

Ross E. The evolving role of antiepileptic drugs in treating neuropathic pain. *Neurology* 2000; 55(5 Suppl 1): S41–6, discussion S54–8.

Rowbotham M, Harden N, Stacey B, Bernstein P, Magnus-Miller L. Gabapentin for the treatment of postherpetic neuralgia: a randomized controlled trial. *Journal of the American Medical Association* 1998; 280: 1837–43.

Rumore M, Schlichting D. Clinical efficacy of antihistaminics as analgesics. *Pain* 1986; 25: 7–22.

Sakurai M, Kanazawa I. Positive symptoms in multiple sclerosis: their treatment with sodium channel blockers, lidocaine and mexiletine. *Journal of Neurological Sciences* 1999; 162: 162–8.

Schnitzer T, Gray W, Paster R, Kamin M. Efficacy of tramadol in treatment of chronic low back pain. *Journal of Rheumatology* 2000; 27: 772–8.

Sindrup S, Jensen T. Pharmacologic treatment of pain in polyneuropathy. *Neurology* 2000; 55: 915–20.

Sindrup S, Andersen G, Madsen C, Smith T, Brosen K, Jensen T. Tramadol relieves pain and allodynia in polyneuropathy: a randomised, double-blind, controlled trial. *Pain* 1999; 83: 85–90.

Taylor P. Cholinergic agonists. In: Gilman A, Rall T, Nies A, Taylor P (eds) *The Pharmacological Basis of Therapeutics*, 8th edn. Pergamon Press, New York, 1990; 122–30.

Tremont-Lukats I, Megeff C, Backonja M. Anticonvulsants for neuropathic pain syndromes: mechanisms of action and place in therapy. *Drugs* 2000; 60: 1029–52.

Wallace M, Magnuson S, Ridgeway B. Efficacy of oral mexiletine for neuropathic pain with allodynia: a double-blind, placebo-controlled crossover study. *Regional Anesthesia and Pain Medicine* 2000; 25: 459–67.

Ward S, Goldberg N, Miller-McCauley V. Pain-related barriers to management of cancer pain. *Pain* 1993; 52: 319–24.

Watson C, Babul N. Efficiency of oxycodone in neuropathic pain: a randomized trial in postherpetic neuralgia. *Neurology* 1998; 50: 1833–41.

Weinbroun A, Rudick V, Paret G, Ben-Abraham R. The role of dextromethorphan in pain control. *Canadian Journal of Anaesthesia* 2000; 47: 585–96.

Wiffen P, Collins S, McQuay H, Carroll D, Jadad A, Moore A. Anticonvulsant drugs for acute and chronic pain. *Cochrane Database System Review* 2000; 3: CD001133.

Index